50 Ways
to Relieve Heartburn, Reflux, and Ulcers

Other books by M. Sara Rosenthal:

The Thyroid Sourcebook
The Gynecological Sourcebook
The Pregnancy Sourcebook
The Fertility Sourcebook
The Breastfeeding Sourcebook
The Breast Sourcebook
The Gastrointestinal Sourcebook
Managing Your Diabetes
Managing Diabetes for Women
The Type 2 Diabetic Woman
The Thyroid Sourcebook for Women
Women & Sadness
Women & Depression
Women & Passion
Women of the '60s Turning 50
50 Ways to Manage Type 2 Diabetes
50 Ways to Prevent Colon Cancer
50 Ways Women Can Prevent Heart Disease

50 *Ways*
to Relieve Heartburn, Reflux, and Ulcers

M. Sara Rosenthal

Foreword by
James Gray, M.D., F.R.C.P.,
Gastroenterologist, Vancouver,
British Columbia

Contemporary Books

Chicago   New York   San Francisco   Lisbon   London   Madrid   Mexico City
Milan   New Delhi   San Juan   Seoul   Singapore   Sydney   Toronto

Library of Congress Cataloging-in-Publication Data

Rosenthal, M. Sara.
    50 Ways to Relieve Heartburn, Reflux, and Ulcers / M. Sara Rosenthal
      p.   cm.
  Includes bibliographical references and index.
  ISBN 0-7373-0472-3 (acid-free paper)
    1. Heartburn—Popular works. 2. Gastroesophageal reflux—Popular
works. 3. Peptic ulcer—Popular works. I. Title: Fifty ways to relieve heartburn,
reflux, and ulcers. II. Title

RC827 .R665   2001
616.3—dc21   00-066001

Contemporary Books

A Division of The McGraw·Hill Companies

1234567890 DOC DOC 0198765432

ISBN 0-7373-0472-3

This book was set in Adobe Cochin and Adobe Futura by Jack Lanning
Printed and bound by R. R. Donnelley & Sons Co.

Cover design by Cheryl Carrington
Illustration on page xv by Elizabeth Weadon Massari
Illustrations on pages 105 and 106 by Ilene Robinette

McGraw-Hill books are available at special quantity discounts to use as
premiums and sales promotions, or for use in corporate training programs.
For more information, please write to the Director of Special Sales, Professional
Publishing, McGraw-Hill, Two Penn Plaza, New York, NY 10121-2298. Or
contact your local bookstore.

The purpose of this book is to educate. It is sold with the understanding that
the publisher and author shall have neither liability nor responsibility for any
injury caused or alleged to be caused directly or indirectly by the information
contained in this book. While every effort has been made to ensure its accuracy,
the book's contents should not be construed as medical advice. Each person's
health needs are unique. To obtain recommendations appropriate to your
particular situation, please consult a qualified health care provider.

This book is printed on acid-free paper.

Contents

Foreword

All of us experience G.I. symptoms to some degree or other during our lives. Many are transient and of little note. Often we know full well that an evening of dietary excess is to blame. But other symptoms are persistent and troublesome, if not worrying. As a result, G.I. symptoms are one of the most frequent complaints heard by family physicians.

The most common of these complaints relate to the upper G.I. tract, including belching, gas, acid, heartburn, and indigestion. Fortunately, most do not represent a serious or life-threatening disease. Determining this, however, requires a careful review of the patient's history and physical examination. This book outlines very clearly the background behind these symptoms, their causes, and the methods used to diagnose and clarify the underlying pathology. It puts the patient or sufferer into the "driver's seat," in beginning treatment as well as in knowing what to expect from health care providers. In addition, we now have a host of treatment options, ranging from lifestyle changes to increasingly varied, specific, and potent drugs, and even surgery. This book clearly spells out therapeutic options and their backgrounds so that an individual can make informed treatment choices. A book such as this represents a great resource for patients and families, as well as for health care providers. After all, being informed and aware is the first, biggest, and most important step in managing and controlling our health.

—James Gray, M.D., F.R.C.P.,
Gastroenterologist, Vancouver,
British Columbia

Acknowledgments

I wish to thank the following people whose expertise and dedication helped to lay so much of the groundwork for this book.

A number of medical advisors on previous works helped me to shape the content for this project. I wish to thank the following people (listed alphabetically): Gillian Arsenault, M.D., C.C.F.P., I.B.L.C., F.R.C.P.; Pamela Craig, M.D., F.A.C.S., Ph.D.; Masood Kahthamee, M.D., F.A.C.O.G.; Gary May, M.D., F.R.C.P.; James McSherry, M.B., Ch.B., F.C.F.P., F.R.C.G.P., F.A.A.F.P., F.A.B.M.P.; Suzanne Pratt, M.D., F.A.C.O.G.; and Robert Volpe, M.D., F.R.C.P., F.A.C.P.

William Harvey, Ph.D., L.L.B., University of Toronto Joint Centre for Bioethics, whose devotion to bioethics has inspired me, continues to support my work and makes it possible for me to have the courage to question and challenge issues in health care and medical ethics. Irving Rootman, Ph.D., Director, University of Toronto Centre for Health Promotion, continues to encourage my interest in primary prevention and health promotion issues.

Larissa Kostoff, my editorial consultant, worked very hard to make this book a reality. And finally, Hudson Perigo, my editor, made many wonderful and thoughtful suggestions to help make this book what it is.

Introduction

How Your G.I. Tract Works

It's difficult to understand how to manage heartburn, reflux, and the range of upper gastrointestinal ailments if you don't understand how the digestive tract works. In fact, it's amazing that anyone feels well after eating, considering how complicated the act of digesting food really is. The term *digesting* refers to the process whereby food is converted into the nutrients we need to live and the waste we don't need. Nutrients are the by-products created when food and drink are broken down into their smallest parts to provide energy to our cells.

The digestive system is a series of tubing, about 22 feet long, that twists and turns from the mouth to the anus. This tubing is lined with mucosa, which contains tiny glands that manufacture digestive juices that break down your food. There are also two other body organs needed for digestion: the liver and the pancreas. Both these organs are responsible for key digestive juices that reach the small intestine through small connecting tubes.

Essentially, the entire digestive tract (or gut) is made up of a series of muscles that are triggered to contract at different stages of digestion. The job of these muscles is to coordinate how and when your food is moved along the tract. Many outside factors can interfere with the muscle coordination of the digestive tract, however. And when that happens, you may not feel well. In fact, more people are hospitalized for gastrointestinal disorders than any other illnesses.

Imagine that your digestive tract is one long subway tunnel with different stops (see Figure I.1). If you were to look at the G.I. "subway map," the first stop is your mouth, the next stop is your pharynx, and the third stop is your esophagus. The esophagus is a major connecting stop. This is where the train stops for a while before switching tracks and moving on to the more active parts of your gut—the stomach, which connects to your duodenum, which connects to your small intestine, which connects to the last stop on the line, your large intestine.

Swallowing your food triggers all the muscles in your digestive tract to begin contracting in wavelike motions known as peristalsis. The act of swallowing is voluntary, but once the food is down the throat, the rest of its movement through the digestive tract is involuntary, or beyond conscious control; at this point, the nervous system takes over. The food goes down the throat into the pharynx and into the esophagus. The esophagus connects the throat to the stomach.

In order for food to get from the esophagus to the stomach, it must go through a crucial tunnel known as the lower esophageal (pronounced eso-fa-jeel) sphincter (LES). This

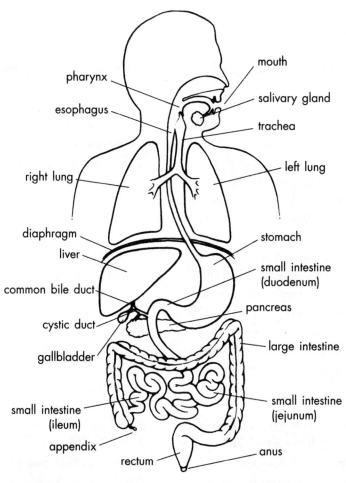

FIGURE I.1 The Gastrointestinal Tract

is a ringlike valve that opens and closes; it's rather like an open piece of tubing that squeezes open and shut to allow food to pass. This sphincter opens and shuts through a series of contractions known as peristalsis, similar to the contractions that occur when you have a bowel movement. These peristaltic "waves," as they're called, come in two stages: primary and secondary. The secondary peristaltic wave is important. This clears away all the trapped food that may have not been cleared in the first or primary wave.

When you swallow food, the LES relaxes to allow the food to pass from the esophagus into the stomach. This prevents digested food from backing up into the esophagus. When the LES isn't working too well, symptoms of gastroesophageal reflux disease (GERD) occur, which include pain, heartburn, bloating, difficulty finishing a meal, stomach discomfort during or after eating (called postprandial discomfort), burping, and the feeling of food coming back up. Often, you'll notice a bitter taste in the back of your throat, and you may also experience gas and/or nausea. (These symptoms are discussed later in the GERD section of this book.)

The stomach is an accordionlike bag of muscle and other tissue near the center of the abdomen just below the rib cage. The bag expands to accommodate food and shrinks when it is empty. The stomach itself is a "holding tank" for food until it can be distributed into more distant parts of the gastrointestinal tract.

In the same way that large coffee grounds remain in the filter, the larger solid particles of food go from the stomach into the duodenum for further digesting, while the mushy, nicely "worked over" food remnants from the stomach quickly pass from the duodenum into the small intestine (midgut, or small bowel). The small intestine is usually called just that, but technically, it is categorized as the duodenum, jejunum, and ileum. For the purposes of this book, I will simply refer to the jejunum and ileum as the small intestine.

What's really happening in digestion is that a series of various tubes along your G.I. tract empty food particles from one into the next. This emptying process is dependent on continuous movement, known as motility, which is controlled by nerves, hormones, and muscles. In fact, if you're experiencing problems in other parts of your body, motility can be slowed down (you'll be constipated and bloated) or speeded up (you'll have diarrhea).

By the time food gets into the small intestine, it is "mushed up" by the digestive secretions of your stomach, pancreas, and biliary tract. This mush stays in the small intestine for a relatively long period of time, and all the usable nutrients are absorbed through the intestinal walls. These nutrients include digested molecules of food, water, and minerals from the diet. The waste products are sent to the large intestine (colon, or large bowel), where they sit around for about a day or two before they are expelled in the form of stools.

This book concentrates on problems north of the colon — that is, everything that usually goes wrong between the esophagus and small intestine. A range of problems can occur here because there are hundreds of nerves and secretions (hormones, enzymes, and chemicals that help to break down food into usable nutrients) that go to work for us whenever we eat. If even one hormone or enzyme is "off" in your system, there will be consequences. G.I. disorders are, themselves, categorized as upper G.I. disorders and lower G.I. disorders. The upper G.I. disorders are the focus of this book and include the following problems.

- Dysmotility: impaired movement of some of the muscles in the G.I. tract. This can lead to a condition known as gastroesophageal reflux disease (GERD), or hypomotility, in which the sphincter at the bottom of the esophagus doesn't contract enough and lets stomach acid come back up. GERD has a number of causes ranging from the unknown (idiopathic) to the overuse of certain drugs. When your G.I. tract is overactive, or hypermotile, you will experience spastic motor disorders because contractions will be much too strong. This causes stomach pain and obstructions throughout your G.I. tract. Treatment for GERD and hypermotility are therefore opposite. Most people suffer from GERD rather than hypermotility.

- Reflux: a fancy word for heartburn; usually a symptom of either GERD or ulcer but could be caused by a perfectly normal occurrence such as pregnancy, for example. This is when your semidigested food comes back up your esophageal sphincter, giving you a bitter taste in your mouth and a burning feeling in your esophagus.

- Ulcer: now known to be caused by a bacteria known as *Helicobacter pylori (H. pylori)*. An ulceration forms on the stomach lining, causing a range of symptoms.

Most of us have experienced a number of minor gastrointestinal upsets in our lifetimes. But this book is about how to manage chronic upper G.I. symptoms, symptoms that are experienced on a regular basis. This can mean a few times a day, a few times a week, or a few times a month. (If you've only experienced the symptoms discussed in this book once in your life, or once a year, you do *not* suffer from chronic gastrointestinal [G.I.] symptoms.) This book gives you the information you need to take control of your symptoms, so you can digest this new century a little better.

PART ONE

Heartburn/Reflux: The First Sign of Trouble

1. What Exactly Is Heartburn/Reflux?

More than sixty-one million American adults experience heartburn about once a month, while another twenty-five million adults suffer from it every day. As mentioned before, food must pass from your esophagus into your stomach through a sphincter known as the lower esophageal sphincter (LES). That sphincter opens and closes through a variety of involuntary muscular contractions known as peristalsis. For a number of reasons, the sphincter doesn't always completely shut after dumping ingested food particles into the stomach. So what happens? The food, now bathed in your stomach acid, comes back up the sphincter, causing a burning sensation in your chest and sometimes a spreading pain throughout your neck and arms that may even be mistaken for a heart attack. You can also experience nausea, belching, and regurgitation of that half-digested food. When it comes back up the sphincter, it doesn't taste as good as it did going down. Thanks to the acid and enzymes to which it's been exposed, the food tastes sour and bitter in your

1

throat. The problem is aggravated when you bend forward or lie down. In fact, you may even find that after an experience like this, you wake up with a sore throat. This problem is clinically called acid reflux and in lay terms is known as heartburn or acid indigestion. For the remainder of this book, the term *heartburn/reflux* will be used.

Heartburn/reflux usually lasts about two hours. Most people find that standing up relieves the burning; that's because gravity helps. You can also take an antacid to clear acid out of the esophagus. Not everyone experiences the same degree of heartburn. Heartburn/reflux can be mild, moderate, or severe. It all depends on why it's occurring, how often it occurs, when it occurs, and how much food backup you have. But for the most part, chronic heartburn/reflux is the first sign of a more serious, underlying health problem.

2. Know the Unusual Symptoms of Heartburn/Reflux

There are a number of atypical or odd symptoms that can suggest you have heartburn/reflux, too, which include:

- Morning hoarseness.
- Drooling.
- Coughing spells.
- Waking up with a sore throat.
- Asthmalike symptoms (or the worsening of asthma symptoms if you are asthmatic). In these cases, you may be having heartburn/reflux at night, which is obstructing your breathing passages, causing all the strange symptoms from coughing to asthma.

It's important to know about unusual symptoms so that you can help your doctor help you—by diagnosing the right problem!

3. Understand the Causes of Heartburn/Reflux

There are several causes of heartburn/reflux. Sometimes a change in diet will make your heartburn/reflux disappear. Classic triggers are chocolate and peppermint, as well as spicy and fatty foods. Citrus foods, including tomatoes and juices, as well as coffee can also trigger an episode of heartburn. Chocolate and peppermint can cause your LES to relax, allowing the stomach contents to back up.

We also know that smoking can relax the LES and cause chronic heartburn. In this case, heartburn symptoms won't go away until you quit smoking or take medication to restore your LES motility.

Sometimes heartburn/reflux is a symptom of an underlying problem, such as gastroesophageal reflux disease (GERD), discussed in Part Three. If this is the case, other symptoms will be associated with your heartburn/reflux, and you will definitely need to alter your lifestyle significantly to correct the problem or take prescription drugs to reduce acid and/or restore your G.I. tract's motility.

A perfectly natural cause of heartburn is pregnancy; in fact, at least 25 percent of all pregnant women suffer from heartburn daily, and 50 percent experience heartburn at some point during their pregnancies. As the uterus expands, it pushes the stomach up against the esophagus, interfering with the LES's proper functioning. In addition, progesterone relaxes muscular contractions, so that the LES doesn't quite close.

For the same reasons pregnancy causes heartburn, so does too much weight in the abdominal region; things get squished in what is already a tight area. Too much weight may push up your stomach and cause your LES to relax.

In infancy, formula feeding can be a cause of heartburn, vomiting, coughing, and failure to thrive. Breastfeeding your infant is the remedy; formula-fed babies are much more prone to gastrointestinal upsets such as heartburn than breastfed babies.

Self-induced Vomiting and G.I. Symptoms

In self-induced vomiting, people cause themselves to vomit on a chronic basis (one to three times per week or more). It's a common feature of the eating disorder bulimia nervosa, which involves bingeing and purging. If you've self-induced vomiting only occasionally due to other circumstances, such as food poisoning, you are not in danger of developing any of these problems.

If you're a chronic purger/vomiter, the first place you'll notice G.I. symptoms is in your mouth. Vomit contains large amounts of stomach acid, which will erode the enamel off your teeth and cause dental problems and cavities. As your teeth become more exposed, you'll start to feel a sensitivity to hot and cold, which can usually be treated by brushing with a toothpaste such as Sensodyne and with a fluoride gel, which can help to protect your teeth from further cavities. Immediately brushing with baking soda and flossing after a vomiting episode is recommended.

You may also notice that about a week after a purging episode, one of your salivary glands, the perotid gland, may swell (known as sialadenosis), which can give you "chip-munk" cheeks. Once you stop vomiting, the glands should go back to their normal size. In the meantime, heat or suck-ing on tart fruits or candies can help.

4. Learn How to Properly Report Your Symptoms

Diagnosing upper G.I. problems usually entails seeing a pri-mary care doctor before a specialist. You want to avoid being misdiagnosed and sent for the wrong series of tests or to the wrong specialist. So, before you report your symptoms to your doctor, remind him or her about all other medical problems you have: allergies, asthma, migraines (often accompanied by nausea), and family history. Chronic prob-lems, such as thyroid disease or diabetes, for example, can definitely affect your digestive system. In addition, other prescription drugs, ranging from antidepressants to non-steroidal anti-inflammatory drugs (NSAIDs) can all affect the G.I. tract. Tell your doctor whether you take aspirin or ibuprofen for commonplace headaches or menstrual cramps. People frequently answer "no" when asked if they're taking medication because they don't realize that this question refers to over-the-counter drugs as well as prescription drugs. And of course, smoking and alcohol can greatly affect your digestive tract, too. Dieting and eating disorders also affect your digestive tract; it's important to reveal all this information.

Tell your doctor what you do for a living. Long commutes and hectic, stressful schedules may indicate unusual eating habits. If you're eating on the run, skipping breakfast, and hitting the couch after work, these practices may contribute to your symptoms.

A Dozen Good Questions

It's important to ask yourself the following before you report your symptoms to your primary care doctor:

1. Do you notice symptoms before or after you eat?
2. Does food seem to aggravate or relieve your symptoms?
3. What are you eating before you notice symptoms?
4. Are you a coffee drinker?
5. Do you consume alcohol?
6. Do you have other symptoms associated with meals, such as early satiety, nausea, vomiting, and so on?
7. Do your symptoms wake you up at night? (Suggests an ulcer.)
8. Does rest seem to help?
9. Does lying down make your symptoms worse?
10. Do you notice any drool when you wake up? (Suggests GERD at night.)
11. Is your voice hoarse when you wake up or do you wake up with a cough? (Suggests reflux at night.)
12. Do you have a sore throat when you wake up? (Suggests reflux at night.)

What Relieves Your Symptoms?

In reporting your symptoms be sure to mention what relieves them. For example, if an over-the-counter antacid helps your symptoms, then it's pretty clear that regardless of whether you have an ulcer or not, you have acidlike dyspepsia (discomfort). If creamy foods relieve your symptoms, then you probably have ulcerlike dyspepsia. If gravity seems to help (standing up versus lying down), combined with antacids, than you have dysmotility-like dyspepsia.

5. Know the Questions Your Doctor Should Ask

When you report chronic heartburn/reflux symptoms, your doctor's questions should include all the dozen questions you ask yourself before you go. Doctors should also ask you the following:

1. How old are you? (Some symptoms are more alarming if you're older than age forty-five.)

2. Have you ever had these symptoms before? (Do you have a past history?)

3. What triggers these symptoms? (Certain foods, timing of meals, and so on.)

4. Have you noticed a worsening of symptoms or do your symptoms appear to be the same?

5. What does your pain feel like (if you have pain)?

6. Do you notice regurgitation (food coming back up) or nausea after a meal? (Indicates a motility disorder.)

7. Do you have difficulty finishing a normal-size meal? (Indicates a motility disorder.)

8. Do you notice any bloating after you eat? (Indicates a motility disorder.)

9. Do you notice hunger pangs throughout the day or at night? (Indicates ulcer.)

10. Do you feel food is sitting in your stomach and not emptying? (Indicates a motility disorder.)

11. How is your appetite? (Helps distinguish whether you answered question 7 consistently.)

12. Are your symptoms worse or better after eating a small meal? (Helps distinguish ulcer from GERD.)

13. How long have you had these symptoms or noticed them? (Why are you here now versus last week?)

14. How do your symptoms relate to other activities (work, exercise, and so on)?

15. What do you do to get relief? (Helps distinguish between ulcer and GERD.)

16. Does belching, passing gas, or having a bowel movement help? (Most people will be embarrassed to say this when answering question 15.)

17. How do you feel when you're standing upright or lifting something? (Is the discomfort posture related? If so, it's probably not an ulcer.)

18. What type of food do you normally eat? (Chocolate, peppermint, fatty foods, and carbonated drinks can all trigger heartburn.)

19. How often do you have a bowel movement? (Are you constipated?)

20. Have you gained weight in the last year or so? (Abdominal weight is often a trigger for GERD.)

6. Know the Difference Between Heartburn and Heart Attack

If you've run to your doctor's office or an emergency room complaining of chest pain after you walk or are physically active, only to find that you have a G.I. problem, you're not alone! Upper G.I. symptoms can cause radiating pains throughout the chest, choking spells, and coughing at night, which could make you think "heart attack." The key question to ask yourself is whether your chest pain is accompanied by:

- Shortness of breath.
- Palpitations.
- Sweating.

If the answer is "no," make sure you report this to your doctor; if your answer is "yes," say so. That could make the difference between a stress test in a cardiologist's office or cutting down on chocolate and peppermint.

7. Know What to Rule Out

Heartburn/reflux symptoms can simply mean that you're suffering from an underlying disorder. Ask your doctor to rule out the following before you're sent home with a diagnosis of simple heartburn/reflux:

- Lactose Intolerance. Over fifty million North Americans suffer from an allergy to milk, known as lactose intolerance. This means that you lack the enzyme lactase, which breaks down the sugar lactose into glucose. Lactose intolerance is extremely common among people of African, Asian, Aboriginal, Mexican, and Jewish descent. With this problem, people experience cramping, gas, bloating, and diarrhea anywhere from fifteen minutes to three hours after eating any dairy product. The treatment is simple: avoid eating dairy products. We can get all the protein and calcium we need from a variety of other foods. If you want to continue to eat dairy foods, however, simply taking Lactaid, which is the enzyme lactase, with your dairy food will enable you to digest it.

- Celiac disease. Celiac is a much rarer, inherited disorder in which one cannot digest an extremely common food substance known as gluten. Gluten is found in wheat, rye, barley, and oats and is in just about every starchy food you can think of. When someone with celiac eats gluten, their intestines can be damaged. Symptoms include severe cramping and a pale or watery stool that often floats in the toilet because the stool contains excess fat that was never absorbed by the body. Celiac is also accompanied by bloating, vomiting, muscle wasting, skin rashes, anemia, and loss of appetite. Early satiety (feeling full after only a few bites of food) is another symptom of celiac disease. Celiac is a "masquerader" disease. People with undiagnosed celiac can be misdiagnosed with GERD. (See Part Three.)

- Other allergies. There are dozens of food allergies that can cause heartburn/reflux, cramping, or diarrhea. Many food allergies cause respiratory symptoms, however. If you find that you experience cramps, gas, or diarrhea after you eat, start keeping a diary and record what you eat so you can isolate the offending food, whether it's dairy or berry.

- Viral infections in the liver. There are three kinds of viral infections to which the liver is vulnerable: hepatitis A, hepatitis B, and hepatitis C. (There are a few more versions of hepatitis, but no blood tests yet to confirm them.) Hepatitis means inflammation of the liver. No matter which type of hepatitis you're infected with, the symptoms are the same, but can take up to 180 days to manifest. During the first phase of hepatitis, symptoms are the worst. You may experience diarrhea, vomiting, fever, nausea, and sometimes skin lesions or joint inflammation. The second phase can cause flulike symptoms, jaundice (yellowing of the skin, because the liver is not processing red blood cells properly), dark urine, and light stools (due to a reduction in bile).

- Cirrhosis of the liver. Cirrhosis is a condition in which the liver becomes scarred by infections, such as hepatitis, or by toxic chemicals. In the Western world, alcoholism causes 75 percent of all cases of cirrhosis. In underdeveloped parts of the world, hepatitis is the major cause of cirrhosis. Cirrhosis is also seen in children, where it is frequently caused by cystic fibrosis or other inherited disorders. Whenever you see the phrase "liver toxicity" as a risk factor from various medications, this refers to the risk of cirrhosis, also known as drug-induced liver toxicity. When a drug enters your bloodstream, your liver converts it into usable chemicals and removes toxins the body cannot use or tolerate. But in the same way a worker can be exposed to toxic fumes (even if it's his job to clean them up), the liver can be overexposed. The more toxins your liver removes, the more damage it incurs. When drugs are damaging your liver, you experience the following symptoms: severe fatigue, abdominal pain and swelling, jaundice (yellow eyes and skin, dark urine), fever, nausea, or vomiting. Liver toxicity can also occur from exposure to environmental toxins, such as benzene (common in many cleaning fluids).

- Gallbladder disease. The gallbladder stores bile for the liver, but you don't really need the gallbladder since the liver is large enough to store as much bile as you'd ever want or need anyway. Nevertheless, we do come equipped with this extra storage space. Bile isn't a very reliable product to store because it can form into little stones inside the gallbladder, known as gallstones (or calculi). Roughly 10 percent of the North American population has gallstones. When the stones become large enough to obstruct the bile ducts, gallbladder disease develops. The symptoms are quite severe; you'll feel sudden, intense pain in the upper abdominal region (which may shoot into your back), sometimes after a fatty meal, but often not related to meals. Vomiting may bring relief although nausea is not a symptom. The pain may then subside over several minutes or hours. Many people mistake gallstone symptoms for heartburn or a heart attack. The obstruction can become infected and even develop gangrene, which is a dire emergency (you don't want gangrene inside your abdominal cavity!). Usually gallbladder disease presents as a series of gallbladder attacks in which you feel pain after meals, and if there's infection, you may experience a fever. The attacks become progressively worse until you decide to have the darned thing removed! As a rule, any abdominal pain accompanied by a fever means serious infection is going on, which is an emergency, warranting emergency medical attention.

- Appendicitis. The appendix (clinically known as the vermiform, or wormlike, appendix) is attached to a section of the colon, and is believed to have played a role in digesting vegetation (such as tree bark or huge leaves) in primitive humans. And who knows? Perhaps if you were stranded in Jurassic Park, and started eating tree bark, your body may even use your appendix. But for now, the appendix serves no known biological purpose. The appendix has a bad habit of becoming infected and inflamed and then bursting, causing the membrane lining the abdominal cavity (the peritoneum) to inflame, called peritonitis. Peritonitis is painful and life-threatening. Just one attack warrants having your appendix surgically removed. The symptoms of appendicitis are two kinds of abdominal pain: severe abdominal pain on your lower right side or a general feeling of abdominal discomfort, resembling gas pains. Diarrhea or a continuous urge to defecate, as well as nausea, vomiting, loss of appetite, and fever are all common symptoms. Symptoms usually develop over six to eighteen hours. If you experience sharp pain on the lower right side, fever of over 101 degrees Fahrenheit, and pain when you move your abdomen or cough or sneeze, it's a sign of rupture. This is an emergency, calling for an emergency appendectomy.

- Pancreatitis. When the bile ducts become blocked (perhaps by gallstones), bile can leak into the pancreas, triggering the enzymes to digest something — except the only thing in the pancreas to digest is the pancreas itself. When pancreatic enzymes attack the pancreas, pancreatitis, or inflammation of the pancreas develops, leading to bleeding, tissue damage, infection, cysts, and even diabetes if the insulin-producing cells are damaged. Pancreatitis can create a big mess, as enzymes and toxins enter your bloodstream and damage other organs. Symptoms are quite severe. Constant abdominal pain travels into the back or through the shoulders. Eating makes the pain worse, and the abdomen feels swollen and tender. Nausea, vomiting, fever, and an increased pulse rate may accompany this pain, and you'll feel—and look—quite sick. Dehydration and low blood pressure happen roughly 20 percent of the time when the kidneys are affected. In short, this is a very severe infection. During an attack, high levels of amylase are found in the blood, as well as abnormal levels of calcium, magnesium, sodium, potassium, and bicarbonate. If the insulin-producing cells are affected, you may also have high blood sugar and high choles-terol levels. But you know what? Pancreatitis will improve on its own. And it's a good thing, too, since there really is no known treatment for acute pancre-atitis, although there are ways to control the damage to other organs caused by the attack.

- Hiatal hernia. When you have a hiatal hernia, stom-ach acid gets into the esophageal opening, causing symptoms of heartburn and reflux. It can be brought on by coughing, vomiting, straining while defecating, or sudden physical exertion. Pregnancy can cause the condition, as well as obesity, and aging is also a factor. Many people over age fifty have small hiatal hernias. Unless you suffer from severe GERD or esophagitis (see Item 22 on page 38), which can complicate a hiatal hernia, you may not require any treatment. If the hernia does cause symptoms, surgery can repair it.

- Peritonitis. Almost any organ in your abdominal region can get infected and inflamed and cause peritonitis, or inflammation of the abdominal wall. Any time you experience abdominal pain and a fever (with or without other symptoms, such as diarrhea or nausea), get yourself to a hospital emergency room for evaluation. Abdominal pain + fever = *major infection*. It could be anything—but it's usually not "nothing." That's the only rule you should remember. Trying to decipher which side your pain is on, or what kind of pain it is (diffuse, acute, severe, really bad, and so on) is a waste of time. The fever tells all.

- Bulimia nervosa. This is an eating disorder that involves self-induced vomiting. Chronic vomiting will also cause GERD, chronic heartburn or sour stomach, and all of the symptoms discussed in Items 1 and 2, as well as sores in the lining of the esophagus, known as Barrett's esophagus (which may cause vomiting of bright red blood). In extreme cases, vomiting can also lead to tears in the mucosal lining of the esophagus, which is a serious condition that will also cause bleeding and vomiting blood. Forceful vomiting can also rupture the esophagus, which is an emergency. Severe chest pain that is brought on by breathing, yawning, or swallowing is a sign of an esophageal rupture.

- Endometriosis. The clinical definition of endometriosis is "abnormal growth of endometrial cells." The endometrium is the lining of the uterus, and endometriosis means that endometrial tissue grows outside the uterus within the general abdominal cavity. Sometimes mild endometriois can cause severe symptoms, while severe endometriosis may cause only mild symptoms. In other words, the severity of your symptoms does not correlate to the severity of the disease. Roughly 5.5 million women in North America have endometriosis. Endometriosis includes so many seemingly unrelated symptoms that it's often missed or just misdiagnosed. Here is a checklist of symptoms you should watch for (there is a sister condition to endometriosis known as adenomyosis, which has similar symptoms). If you find you have at least two of these symptoms during your period or even chronically, you may want to be checked out for endometriosis:

- Pelvic pain and/or painful intercourse. (In one survey, 78 percent of women with endometriosis reported pain severe enough to wake them up at night or interfere with their falling asleep.)
- Infertility. (This is often the only symptom women experience—even with advanced cancer.)
- Abnormal cycles or periods.
- Nausea and/or vomiting.
- Exhaustion.
- Bladder problems.
- Frequent infections.
- Dizziness.
- Painful defecation.
- Lower backaches.
- Irritable bowels (loose, watery, and often bloody diarrhea). Many women with irritable bowel disease (IBS) really have endometriosis.
- Other stomach problems.
- Low-grade fever.

• Ovarian cancer symptoms. A book on G.I. disorders
  may be a more appropriate place to discuss ovarian
  cancer than a book on women's health. That's because
  the symptoms of ovarian cancer are G.I.—not gynecological. This is a deadly cancer for women because
  70 percent of it is found in an advanced stage. Why is
  that? Because the symptoms are so vague and gastrointestinal in nature that few women suspect it's cancer at all—let alone a gynecological cancer. If discovered
  early, however, ovarian cancer carries an 85 to 95 percent five-year survival rate. Going for regular pelvic
  exams and watching for the following G.I. symptoms
  will help you catch this cancer before it's too late.

  · Symptoms of GERD (heartburn, bloating, feel-
    ing full early in the meal, gas, and other
    symptoms discussed in Item 22 on page 38).

  · Discomfort in the lower abdomen.

  · Painless swelling or bloating in the lower
    abdomen.

  · Loss of appetite.

  · Gas and indigestion.

  · Nausea.

  · Weight loss.

  · Constipation.

  · Pain during intercourse.

  These symptoms are particularly alarming when you
  have:

  · A family history of breast, ovarian, or colorectal
    cancer.

- Never been pregnant.
- Taken fertility drugs in the past.
- Been exposed to environmental toxins.
- Had irregular periods.
- A high-fat, low-fiber diet.

If you have two or more of these symptoms, go to your doctor and say, "I want you to feel for an enlarged ovary or mass." If this doesn't reveal anything, ask if you can have a ruling-out transvaginal pelvic ultrasound so you can be sure. When it comes to this kind of deadly cancer, better safe than sorry. If your doctor gives you a hard time, tell him or her that you don't want to be another ovarian cancer statistic —or blame this book for your overcaution! For more information, consult my book *The Gynecological Sourcebook*.

- Myobacterium aviumintracellular complex (MAC). This is only something to rule out if you are HIV-positive. MAC is really an atypical form of tuberculosis, which doesn't develop until you are in an advanced stage of AIDS, in which your T-cells are fewer than fifty. In this case, the cough is less severe, but you will suffer from severe gastrointestinal symptoms. Symptoms of MAC include weight loss, chronic high fever, severe anemia, chills and night sweats, abdominal pain, chronic diarrhea, swollen lymph nodes, reduction in white blood cells (neutropenia), and an enlarged liver and spleen.

8. Know the Red-Flag Symptoms

There are certain red-flag symptoms that warrant an immediate investigation by a gastrointestinal specialist; these doctors are called gastroenterologists. Alarming symptoms don't necessarily mean you have something serious; they mean you should rule out something serious. The word that characterizes alarming symptoms from chronic symptoms is *sudden*. If you're between the ages of forty-five and fifty-five, and you suddenly notice the onset of any of the following symptoms, don't wait and see what happens. Get yourself to a doctor's office as soon as possible, where you can be referred for testing or to a gastroenterologist.

Symptoms that indicate a possible serious illness, such as cancer, include:

- Weight loss. (You've lost at least 5 to 10 pounds in the last month without trying.)
- Vomiting (particularly vomiting blood).
- Bloody saliva.
- Black stool or bloody stool. (Black stools mean blood is in your stools.)
- Anemia. (This could mean that you're bleeding from your gastrointestinal tract.)
- Persistent abdominal pain. (Nothing makes it go away.)
- New and unusual symptoms. (Particularly if you're between ages forty-five to fifty or over age sixty-five.)
- Food or liquid sticks in your throat. (Called dysphagia, or difficulty swallowing.)
- Feeling full after a few bites. (If it's accompanied by heartburn, pain, bloating, and nausea, it's likely

GERD or a motility disorder, but this is an alarming symptom nonetheless.)

If your doctor has prescribed medication for your G.I. symptoms and you're not responding to it or getting better that's another alarm sign. In this case, it could simply be that the wrong diagnosis was made. It could also mean that there is a more serious, underlying disease at work, which you need to have evaluated as soon as possible.

9. Know the Right Diagnostic Tests

If your doctor determines your symptoms are related to acid/ulcer, reflux, or dysmotility (which is part of GERD), then there's probably no reason to get further tests, and he can treat you with lifestyle/diet counseling (see Part Five) or medication (see Part Four). But if you have alarming symptoms, discussed in Item 8, or there is some confusion about what you have, then it's probably a good idea to go to a gastroenterologist for an evaluation, who in turn may send you for tests to rule out or confirm various diagnoses.

These tests can include:

- An upper G.I. series. This means that the doctor takes a series of X-ray images followed by a barium tracer, so she can get a picture of what's going on in your upper G.I. tract. This should be the first step. X-rays of the esophagus, stomach, and duodenum will rule out an ulcer, but they won't tell you anything about acid or motility. Your doctor can get some information about how the esophagus contracts, and she can tell if there's any decreased activity in elderly patients or in people with diabetes. But unless you have really severe gastric discomfort, for example, leftover food particles in your stomach, these tests won't tell you much about motility.

- Endoscopy. Here, a thin, lighted tube is passed down your esophagus. If you have chronic heartburn, this test will tell your doctor whether your heartburn has caused esophagitis (inflammation of the tissue lining the esophagus). If your heartburn is bad enough to cause inflammation, the doctor will likely treat it with a strong antacid drug, such as an H2 receptor antagonist. Over-the-counter antacids probably aren't strong enough in this case.

- Biopsy. This shouldn't be necessary unless you have confusing results from your endoscopy, coupled with alarming symptoms. In this case, a tiny piece of tissue that lines your esophagus is removed for investigation.

- The Bernstein test. In this test, a mild acid is dripped through a tube that's placed about midway in your esophagus. This test confirms whether your symptoms are a result of contact between your esophageal lining and acid. It isn't usually necessary if a good history is done.

- Scintigraphy. This gastric emptying test, involves nuclear medicine. Eggs are scrambled with technetium, a radioactive substance. You swallow the eggs and a gamma counter determines how quickly the eggs empty out of the stomach.

- Esophageal manometry. This test measures the pressure or tension of liquids in your esophagus. This is best for people with atypical symptoms or those with difficulty swallowing.

- pH Testing. If your doctor is still confused, the acid levels inside your esophagus can be measured through pH testing.

10. Understand the Treatment for Heartburn/Reflux Is Usually Diagnosis

Roughly 40 to 60 percent of all people with heartburn symptoms seem to do well with modifying their lifestyles (see Part Five) and taking over-the-counter antacids when needed. Nonprescription antacids provide temporary relief only and should not be considered first-line therapies unless you have only occasional symptoms. As discussed in Part Four, using these antacids for long periods of time (longer than two to three weeks) can cause problems, including diarrhea, as well as too much calcium or magnesium in your system.

Remember, heartburn/reflux is often the first sign of a more serious, underlying problem, and treatment can include prescription drugs or even antibiotics if an ulcer is suspected.

PART TWO

Diagnosing and Managing Ulcers

11. Understand What an Ulcer Is

The word *ulcer* means that a small area of an organ or tissue has sloughed off, resulting in a sore. Dozens of types of ulcers can occur in the human body; only about 20 percent of all ulcers are, in fact, ulcers in the gastrointestinal tract. Here, a small part of the lining of the duodenum (in about 90 percent of the cases), esophagus (about 5 percent of the time, known as Barrett's esophagus), or the stomach itself (called a gastric ulcer, from the Greek *gaster*, which also occurs about 5 percent of time) has somehow worn away. It is estimated that one in ten Americans develops an ulcer at some time. Of those, three have duodenal ulcers for every one with a gastric ulcer.

Once food reaches the stomach (assuming it doesn't come back up the esophagus), it's ground up by forceful contractions of the stomach muscles and then mixed with acid and the enzyme pepsin. Your stomach lining is made of a tough material that can withstand the acid and pepsin, which are powerful enough to liquefy a piece of meat. If just a tiny portion of your stomach's lining wears away, however, you'll feel pain at that spot from the acid and pepsin. This is why ulcers are sometimes known as peptic ulcer disease.

It's also important to understand the shape and size of ulcers. When you get a blister on your foot from new shoes, the blister itself is very tender, forming a deep cavity, and the area around the blister becomes red and inflamed. Same thing here: when something wears down the lining of your duodenum, a blister or ulcer forms, which is often 1 to 2 inches wide and surrounded by an inflamed area. This inflamed area is known as an ulcer crater.

As mentioned above, about 90 percent of all ulcers form in the duodenum. You may be told you have a duodenal ulcer instead of a peptic ulcer; but they're the same thing. Duodenal ulcers are usually smaller than ulcers in the stomach or esophagus and tend to heal faster.

12. Understand the Real Causes of Ulcers

As recently as the 1970s and 1980s, ulcers were considered chronic conditions that required the ulcer sufferer to eat bland foods and take antacids with milk. Most of us recall only male relatives with ulcers, our fathers, uncles, or grandfathers; that's because ulcers tend to affect men (aged forty-five to sixty-five) about twice as often as women. It was presumed that because men don't express their emotions as freely as women, bottled-up emotions and stress caused ulcers to form. This doesn't sound all that illogical, given that we do tend to make more hydrochloric acid when we're upset or under stress. Nevertheless, this explanation has been proven wrong.

Ulcers are now believed to be caused by a bacterial infection called *Helicobacter pylori (H. pylori)*. When the infection is treated with antibiotics, the ulcer goes away forever. As we age, we are more likely to have *H. pylori* in our bodies. The incidence rate *is* age related. At age twenty-five, you have a 25 percent chance of having *H. pylori;* at age fifty, you have a 50 percent chance of having *H. pylori.* Ulcers affect more men than women for reasons that aren't known. Experts muse whether estrogen and progesterone somehow protect women from ulcers, but no clear research shows why ulcers tend to favor the male body over the female body. (Certainly dozens of other conditions affect more women than men, which we also can't explain.) *H. pylori* incidence is equal among men and women, but fewer women with the bacteria than men develop ulcers.

Studies show that *H. pylori* infects over 90 percent of all people with duodenal ulcers, and over 70 percent of those with gastric ulcers. (This is discussed in more detail toward the end of this chapter.) The theory is that *H. pylori* weakens the lining of the G.I. tract, making it easier for acid or other agents to wear down the lining. That said, millions of people are walking around with *H. pylori* who will never develop an ulcer. So, why is *H. pylori* more potent in some people than others? No one is sure, but it's very likely that when combined with another trigger, such as certain irritating medications, smoking, or even a genetic predisposition to ulcers (studies show that ulcers do run in families), it will become active. It's like what happens when you use two ingredients in baking; alone, both ingredients do nothing to make a cake rise, but when they are combined, the cake rises beautifully.

13. Know Who Is Infected with *H. Pylori*

Half the world is infected with *H. pylori*! In the United States, that translates into about forty million people, out of whom 10 to 20 percent will develop ulcers. People who live together or who share close quarters are more vulnerable to *H. pylori* infection for the same reasons they catch various flu viruses or colds. People who sneeze, cough, and kiss together may have ulcers in common. In fact, it's been well known since the 1950s that family members of ulcer patients are three times more likely to develop ulcers than those in the general population.

History even records ulcer outbreaks similar to influenza outbreaks in various neighborhoods. A famous outbreak happened during the London bombings in World War II; stress was blamed for the outbreak at the time.

Perhaps one of the most important groups found to have *H. pylori* were those with some types of stomach cancer. In fact, *H. pylori* infection may triple your risk of developing certain stomach cancers (usually uncommon) even if no ulcers are present.

14. Know the Symptoms That Spell U-L-C-E-R

It's possible to have an ulcer without knowing about it because ulcers don't always cause symptoms. If you do have a symptom, it's usually a localized pain in the upper G.I. tract area. Many people find that this pain resembles a hunger pang that often wakes them up at night. The pain may be partially or completely relieved by eating food or by taking antacids. Ulcer pain is usually worse on an empty stomach. Classic ulcer pain tends to strike late in the morning, late in the afternoon, and about 3 o'clock in the morning. Eating food helps because it buffers the acid (as do antacids).

In general, any stomach pain that is strong enough to wake you up is likely to be an ulcer because the G.I. tract "goes to sleep" at night when you do and usually only wakes up when you do, too. That's why that morning bowel movement is like the "rooster crow" for many people. If you were to define the severity of the pain on a 1-to-5 scale, you'd probably rate this pain as a 2 or 3.

Less Common Symptoms

Nausea, vomiting (sometimes vomiting blood; sometimes throwing up a meal you ate two days ago), no appetite, and weight loss can accompany your pain. You may also notice that your stools are blacker than normal or tarry (this indicates that there is blood in the stools), or that they have a foul odor (fouler than usual, that is). Some of the symptoms of ulcers are on the red-flag list in the previous chapter; that's because once an ulcer has developed, it's important to treat it before it gets worse. Other ulcer symptoms include dizziness, weakness, or paleness (a sign of anemia) and severe back pain (your pain is traveling).

15. Know the Other Causes of Ulcers

In the absence of *H. pylori*, there are some other causes of ulcers. For example, the resistance of your stomach lining to acid and pepsin is lowered when you regularly take aspirin or other nonsteroidal anti-inflammatory drugs (NSAIDs), ranging from ibuprofen to Naprosyn. NSAIDs have been shown in one study to suppress the growth of malignant cells in the colon. (In fact, coffee and NSAIDs taken together reinforce the suppression.) Nevertheless, if NSAIDs are the reason you have an ulcer, you need to weigh their obvious detriment against the benefit shown by this particular study.

Alcohol can definitely lower the resistance of the stomach lining to acid and pepsin. That includes the alcohol in various medications. Smoking can wear down the stomach lining. Smokers are 50 percent more likely to develop stomach or duodenal ulcers as nonsmokers. Ulcers also take longer to heal in smokers.

Research shows that in people with poor motility, substances that normally belong in the small intestine sometimes back up into the stomach. These substances can include harmful bacteria other than *H. pylori*, which can also wear down the stomach lining.

Sometimes your family can wear down your stomach lining. Studies show that if a family member develops a gastric or duodenal ulcer, you're likely to as well. At one point, it was thought that there was a genetic predisposition to having less resistant or "thinner" stomach linings. It's more likely that family members infect one another with *H. pylori*, and that's why ulcers run in families. Similarly, colds and flus will attack a household.

Age is also a factor in ulcers. Ulcers tend to occur after age forty-five, especially in men. Again, there's no clear reason why ulcers favor men over women, but more men do take aspirin as a blood thinner than women, and men tend to drink more alcohol, too.

What About Stress?

The more stress you're under, the more likely you are to take aspirin and ibuprofen because you may find you get stress-related headaches. It's also known that you produce more hydrochloric acid when you're under stress. The problem is that ulcers are not caused by excess acid; they're caused by a worn-down stomach lining. In fact, some researchers believe that both too much or too little acid and pepsin can lead to an ulcer.

If you take aspirin, you're more likely to develop a stomach or gastric ulcer than a duodenal ulcer—especially if you take more than four aspirins per week for a period of three months. The flip side is that many people take aspirin as a blood thinner to lower their risk of cardiovascular problems. Again, you need to weigh your ulcer against your risk of cardiovascular disease. (Better yet, why don't you just change your diet and cut out the aspirin! See Part Five.)

Ulcers in the Esophagus

The causes for ulcers in the esophagus are related to heartburn and reflux. The esophagus wasn't meant to contain acid. Therefore, if you're suffering from heartburn/reflux (see Part One) or gastroesphageal reflux disease (see Part Three), then severe reflux could be bad enough to cause an ulcer in your esophagus. In this case, your ulcer is caused by acid in an area where it doesn't belong. *H. pylori* is not considered a culprit in these kinds of ulcers. Only about 5 percent of all ulcers will be this type.

16. Understand How Doctors Diagnose Ulcers

In the previous section on heartburn, I devoted considerable space to how to report your G.I symptoms to your doctor. All those questions regarding how your symptoms relate to food will tell your doctor whether you have an ulcer or not. Doctors categorize upper G.I. patients into those with ulcer symptoms and those with non-ulcer symptoms. Ulcer symptoms are often obvious. Most gastroenterologists, for example, will be able to diagnose an ulcer based on the answers to a few good questions. Then, they'll follow up on their ulcer hunch by screening for *H. pylori* infection using a breath test. (*H. pylori* can also be found with a blood test.) If you test positive for *H. pylori*, you'll be treated with antibiotics as well as an H2 (histamine type 2) receptor antagonist (H2 blocker), such as cimetidine or ranitidine (discussed more in Part Four). Some doctors may narrow down the diagnosis by treating you with an H2 receptor antagonist, which should work if, in fact, you have an ulcer. Then, if you don't get better, your doctor will try a different drug. Although this philosophy sounds somewhat half baked, it's actually a good management approach for G.I. therapy. In short, an H2 receptor drug can sort out whether or not you have an ulcer because you'll either get better, or you won't.

17. Know When Ulcers Are Emergencies

You've probably heard about ulcers "punching a hole through your stomach." Well, this can happen in rare and severe situations. In this case, the ulcer can furrow beyond the lining of the stomach or duodenum into the actual wall that separates the stomach or duodenum from the rest of your abdominal cavity, causing G.I. bleeding. Symptoms include dizziness, weakness, and paleness (all due to anemia), vomiting of blood, and passing black or foul-smelling stools. If the ulcer goes beyond the stomach wall, the stomach acid and other juices can get into your abdominal cavity, which requires emergency treatment. You'll be in a lot of pain and will probably need surgery to repair the hole or perforation. Sometimes an ulcer that perforates the wall of the stomach or duodenum is a sign of an ulcerating tumor, not a usual stomach ulcer.

An ulcer can also block important pathways your food needs to go through to be digested. This is a pretty rare event, but the symptoms include vomiting up food you ate days ago while your stomach pain spreads throughout your abdominal cavity. This is another case when surgery may be necessary.

18. Know the Treatment for Ulcers

If you have an ulcer, and test positive for the *H. pylori* bacteria, treating the ulcer involves triple therapy. This involves a combination of two antibiotics and the antacid bismuth (Pepto Bismol), which are prescribed together. It's believed that *H. pylori* has a variety of strains. Using two antibiotic agents improves the chances that the right strain of *H. pylori* will be killed. Researchers have found that metronidazole and tetracycline work well, unless you have taken metronidazole before. In that case, clarithromycin is substituted for metronidazole.

If your ulcer is actively "in flare," you'll probably be prescribed an H2 receptor drug or a proton pump inhibitor (see Part Four) as well as metronidazole, amoxicillin, or clarithromycin.

Once you're treated for an ulcer, it's important to see your doctor six to eight weeks after your ulcer has healed to make sure that you are, indeed, ulcer free. It's also important to make sure that what you had was in fact an ulcer and not a cancerous lesion. Cancer can sometimes be mistaken for an ulcer.

19. Know the Right Way to Take Antibiotics

In hospitals all over the world, we're seeing mutated bacteria that nothing can touch. The Centers for Disease Control estimate that about forty thousand Americans die each year due to antibiotic-resistant strains of bacteria. The biggest problem is that people don't understand how antibiotics work, and therefore stop taking them as soon as they feel well. This doesn't let the antibiotic kill the bacteria it was meant to kill, and allows the bacteria time to mutate and resist that antibiotic.

Shockingly, more than 50 percent of people in one survey failed to take their antibiotics as prescribed—even though 75 percent of those surveyed said that they were counseled about how to take their medication.Therefore, it's crucial that you follow these directions when an antibiotic is prescribed for treating your ulcer (or for any other reason):

- Take your antibiotic as prescribed (with meals, at night, or whenever). Don't take four pills a day when you're supposed to take one; don't take the drug once a day when you're supposed to take it three times a day. In other words, be sure you understand how many pills to take in a day and when to take them. Skipping doses can allow the antibiotic to become ineffective and give the bacteria time to mutate. Doubling up on a dose is usually not encouraged, either.

- Ask how alcohol, milk, or other foods affect the antibiotic. Some foods can weaken the antibiotic and make it ineffective.

- *Finish the bottle.* Don't stop taking the antibiotic because you feel better. You're feeling better because the bacteria may be dying; but they're not dead until the bottle is finished. Many antibiotics must be taken several times a day for ten or more days to do the job, even though you will probably feel better within forty-eight hours.

- Never take leftover antibiotics from the bottle you didn't finish last year, and never borrow an antibiotic from your sister-in-law's friend's mother, or lend it to your brother's friend's sister-in-law!

- Be prepared for some side effects. Antibiotics kill off friendly bacteria in your body, too, and can cause vaginal yeast infections. You may also experience nausea, diarrhea, rashes, or a number of other side effects. Ask your doctor what to expect before you fill your prescription. Antibiotics may also affect other medications you're taking and render them ineffective. Oral contraceptives and antibiotics don't mix; for example, you may wind up trading an ulcer for a baby if you're not careful.

20. Know If You Should Be Screened for *H. Pylori*

By understanding that the bacteria *H. pylori* is the chief cause of ulcers, we now know how to prevent an ulcer from coming back or reforming after it was previously treated. The presence of *H. pylori* + a past history of ulcer = *new ulcer*. So unless *H. pylori* is eradicated, the rate of ulcer recurrence is 60 to 80 percent in the first year without any other therapy.

So one good question is, Shouldn't everyone be screened for *H. pylori*? No; many people will test positive for *H. pylori*, but only a few of us will ever develop ulcers. Screening and treating everybody for *H. pylori* infection is not only impractical, but no health care system could possibly afford it. In the United States, imagine how much money it would cost to screen the entire population and treat the forty million people with *H. pylori* with not one but two and sometimes three kinds of antibiotics! This would amount to billions of dollars.

The only people who need to be treated for *H. pylori* infection are those who have ulcers or selected people who have chronic non-ulcer pain; new studies found that this group seemed to benefit from *H. pylori* treatment, too (see Table 20.1). But for the most part, people with other G.I. disorders, ranging from GERD to appendicitis, don't need to think about *H. pylori*. It's generally just an "ulcer thing."

Researchers believe that different strains of *H. pylori*, as well as secondary factors, that combine with *H. pylori* to trigger an ulcer. For example, John may take aspirin, NSAIDs, drink, or smoke; Bill may be into living organically and never put an impure thing in his body—be it medication or cigarettes. Both Bill and John can be infected

Table 20.1 Who Should Be Treated for *H. Pylori*?

If You Have	And Are *H. Pylori* Positive
No ulcer	No
Non-ulcer dyspepsia	Sometimes
Gastric ulcer	Yes
Duodenal ulcer	Yes

with *H. pylori,* but John is far more likely to develop an ulcer than Bill.

The strongest evidence that suggests *H. pylori* causes ulcers is that ulcers don't come back when *H. pylori* is treated. There is also an ethical issue regarding treating asymptomatic people with antibiotics. Since antibiotics can lead to resistant strains of bacteria, discussed in Item 19, widespread antibiotic therapy can be harmful to the general public.

PART THREE

Non-Ulcer Symptoms and GERD

(Gastroesophageal Reflux Disease)

21. Understand NUD

You may be a real "NUD case." And in G.I. language, that's not an insult, or even a left-handed compliment. It means that your doctor has diagnosed you with non-ulcer dyspepsia, or rather, "stomach pain and discomfort not due to ulcer." Sorry to be so vague, but NUD simply means that your pain and heartburn symptoms do not sound like an ulcer. NUD is not a disease; it is an umbrella term that helps doctors distinguish their ulcer patients from their non-ulcer patients. When a doctor tells you that you have NUD, it's like telling a person with a runny nose and tearing eyes that her symptoms are due to "noncold virus discomfort" when, in fact, she has an allergy. In other words, it sounds medical but it is not a clear-cut diagnosis that should satisfy you. When you have NUD, your discomfort is probably due to two things: gastroesophageal reflux disease (GERD) or dysmotility (meaning "gastrointestinal tract muscles not moving very well").

Gastroenterologists explain the typical NUD patient as someone who has symptoms that are completely indistinguishable from someone who has ulcers and heartburn but whose stomach and esophagus look completely normal in diagnostic tests. In these cases, it's believed that there is an underlying disorder at work called dysmotility, in which the muscles of the G.I. tract are not as coordinated as they should be.

Symptoms of NUD can, in fact, be so vague that many doctors essentially flip a coin to decide what to rule out by prescribing a short course of drug therapy to see what happens. In other words, people with NUD will either respond to a particular medication or not; the response will tell the doctor whether that person has GERD or dysmotility, or both.

The most logical question to ask your doctor when you are told you have NUD is whether the acid problem you may have is too much acid in the wrong place. Acid in the wrong place points to dysmotility. (See Item 23.)

22. Understand GERD

GERD is a confusing disease comprised of chronic heartburn/reflux (see Part One), as well as many of the dysmotility symptoms in Item 23 (bloating, nausea, and so on). One survey showed that 75 percent of people suffering from non-ulcer pain and heartburn have additional symptoms. In this case, reflux is caused when the lower esophageal sphincter (LES)—the muscle connecting the esophagus with the stomach—doesn't close properly after the food passes from the esophagus to the stomach. So acid-laced food comes back up.

In the medical community, GERD is referred to as an "iceberg" disease in that there are many symptoms at the base common to all people with GERD. As the iceberg narrows into various jagged peaks, symptoms vary. For example, all people will have reflux, but not all people will feel burning or bloating or nausea. On the other hand, some people may experience every imaginable symptom of GERD and dysmotility. Moreover, the severity of the symptoms differs, which can depend on how severe LES dysfunction is, how much fluid is coming up from the stomach, and even how effective saliva is at neutralizing the reflux. Most experts today classify GERD as both an acid problem, in that acid is in the wrong part of your G.I. tract, and a motility problem.

Severe GERD can cause inflammation of the esophageal lining, known as esophagitis. This can lead to narrowing of the esophagus. Severe GERD can also cause an ulcer.

Pregnancy and GERD

In pregnancy the smooth muscle relaxes to prevent the uterus from contracting during the nine months of pregnancy. Unfortunately, this can create a number of gastrointestinal symptoms, including GERD. In this case, your expanding uterus presses up against your esophagus, interfering with the lower esophageal sphincter and causing heartburn. If you've suffered from GERD in the past, pregnancy often makes it worse. Morning sickness can also cause nausea and reflux, and many women will also be plagued with anal symptoms, such as hemorrhoids. Treatment for G.I. symptoms during pregnancy is tea and sympathy. Various herbal teas may help relieve certain symptoms, but beyond that, taking any sort of medication during pregnancy is not recommended without strict permission from your doctor. For more information on pregnancy symptoms, consult my book *The Pregnancy Sourcebook*.

23. Understand Dysmotility

Dysmotility means "things not moving well." Food travels from the esophagus into the stomach, which slowly releases it into the small intestine. There can be problems on any or all "floors" of this elevator. Things can get stuck between the esophagus and stomach, causing the classic GERD symptoms of heartburn and reflux. In this case, the lower esophageal sphincter relaxes when it should be taut, allowing food to come back up. Or, food can get stuck between the stomach and small intestine, which causes symptoms of bloating, fullness, and so on. People with dysmotility will find that most diagnostic tests will come back normal; the diagnostic tests available for G.I. disorders are generally for the purpose of ruling out an ulcer, tumor, or inflammation.

Dysmotility, with all its varying symptoms, is typically a chronic condition. Symptoms keep coming back, and by the time dysmotility is finally diagnosed, most people have had these symptoms for a long time. The only way you can stop symptoms from recurring is by changing your lifestyle habits or taking a motility drug as a maintenance therapy. The classic case of dysmotility goes something like this: You may notice that you suffer from chronic gas, bloating, and feeling full despite your efforts to control the symptoms. You may also have a lot of stress combined with poor eating habits. Your doctor prescribed an H2 receptor antagonist (Tagamet), but it didn't help. You were then sent for tests, which always come back normal. You were also counseled about changing your diet and lifestyle to avoid symptoms, but you're not very good at making dietary changes. Your symptoms persist, and you're miserable. Several months later, another doctor, perhaps a G.I. specialist, diagnoses a motility disorder, prescribes a specific motility drug or prokinetic agent (promovement drug), and your symptoms begin to disappear.

Dysmotility is often missed because doctors tend to think "ulcers" or "reflux" when they're diagnosing upper G.I. disorders. Dysmotility is one of those conditions that is a little "outside the box." Many times, lesser symptoms such as gas or bloating are not reported either.

When Dysmotility Is a Symptom of Another Disease

There are many disorders that can cause dysmotility symptoms. Reviewing this list might be a good way to rule out some underlying causes for your G.I. symptoms:

- Anorexia nervosa. This eating disorder involves refusal of food (starvation). When it comes to G.I. symptoms, people with anorexia nervosa will experience symptoms of dysmotility: feeling full after eating a few bites, abdominal fullness and bloating, gas, nausea, and possibly heartburn from poor functioning of the lower esophageal sphincter. Starvation causes the G.I. tract to slow down, causing a real, physical problem of dysmotility. The treatment in this case is the same as that used for anyone with dysmotility. Some complications arise, however, when people don't believe that anorexics are truly suffering from the dysmotility symptoms they describe. It is common for symptoms to be misconstrued as the psychological element of the disease. In other words, others think you're saying, "I'm full," or "I don't feel well" because you're afraid of the food, not because there are really organic symptoms at work that delay gastric emptying and cause your symptoms. If you have dysmotility symptoms and are not being believed, insist on a referral to a gastroenterologist and tell your eating disorder specialist(s), "I'm not making this up just to avoid eating; in fact, I'm disclosing these symptoms to you so I can begin to recover and eat normal amounts of food comfortably. I believe I'm suffering from a motility problem, which I understand is a physical manifestation of my eating disorder." That ought to do the trick and get you the treatment you need.

- Bulimia nervosa. As discussed in Item 7, bulimia is an eating disorder characterized by purging, usually in the form of self-induced vomiting. But it can also involve abusing laxatives and/or diuretics; misusing other drugs, including thyroid medication or insulin (Type 1 diabetic women may deliberately withhold their insulin to induce weight loss), or overexercising. Regardless of the purge method used, the binge episode by itself can distend the abdomen, causing breathlessness, as your bloated stomach presses against your diaphragm. There are even documented cases of people requiring emergency surgery as a result of tears in the stomach wall due to overstretching.

24. Ask About Prokinetic Drugs

Most gastroenterologists agree that making certain lifestyle adjustments can probably clear up GERD and restore motility without the use of drug therapy. See Part Five for details.

Otherwise, if you suffer from bloating, feeling full, and the other symptoms of dysmotility, along with your heartburn and pain, then you don't need an acid-suppressing drug or an H2 receptor antagonist (H2 blocker). What you need is a prokinetic drug that will improve motility and get things moving again. A prokinetic drug regulates the muscles in your G.I. tract by telling your brain to send the right messages to the muscles that control the G.I. tract. Those muscles include the lower esophageal sphincter, which will stop relaxing when it should be contracting. In essence, a prokinetic drug helps your food get from the esophagus into the stomach and then from the stomach into the small intestine. It does this by improving LES pressure and peristalsis, which gets rid of the acid in the esophagus and improves gastric emptying. Once that happens, you'll notice that all those symptoms caused by food sitting in your stomach too long will disappear.

25. Know When *Not* to Use Acid Suppressants

Only 5 to 10 percent of all GERD sufferers are in fact secreting too much stomach acid. Once that lower esophageal sphincter delivers the food into the stomach and squeezes shut like it's supposed to, acid-laced food will no longer come back up into your esophagus. No more half-digested food, no more reflux or heartburn, and therefore, no more need to use antacids or H2 receptor antagonists.

In cases in which you have severe reflux that has caused esophagitis or an ulcer, an H2 receptor drug, such as cimetidine, famotidine, nizatidine, or ranitidine, can help to alleviate your acid symptoms until the prokinetic drug starts to work its magic. Many doctors in this case will instead prescribe one of the proton pump inhibitors, such as omeprazole, which inhibits an enzyme necessary for acid secretion.

If you have only mild reflux, even regular over-the-counter antacids, combined with prokinetic drugs, may help. In most cases of GERD, however, the acid is simply in the wrong spot—something an acid-lowering drug cannot do much about. (More information about these drugs is discussed in Part Four.)

26. Further Tests for NUD and GERD Symptoms

If you have symptoms of dysmotility and GERD and are not getting better with cisapride alone or in combination with other drugs, that's alarming. In this case, your doctor should investigate why you're not getting better by doing further diagnostic tests.

An upper G.I. series can shed some light on what's going on in your esophagus with swallowing, as well as how well your stomach is emptying. The scrambled egg test, mentioned in Part One, can also help to document the time it takes for the esophagus to clear the tracer out, which will help your doctor to understand a little more about esophageal clearing. This test may also provide information on how quickly your stomach empties both solids and liquids.

As described earlier, this test is done using nuclear medicine. A nuclear medicine technician will play "chef," and sit down in the laboratory with a frying pan and make you scrambled eggs with technetium as a tracer. You'll eat the eggs, then a gamma counter will be placed over your stomach after you've swallowed to follow the eggs on their journey through your G.I. tract. The test will determine how quickly the eggs leave your stomach. This test should only be done once ulcers, esophagitis, or tumors have been ruled out through endoscopy.

Many gastroenterologists believe, however, that there are no good tests to check gastric emptying or motility. If your gastroenterologist comes from this school, then she may decide to try a combination of drugs to see how well you respond. Atypical symptoms may warrant pH testing or manometry, discussed in Part One.

Certain tests need to be done properly to extract any useful information. For example, people who have difficulty swallowing need to be investigated for some sort of obstacle or obstruction in the esophagus. In this case, imaging tests need to be performed while you're in various positions, when the most stress is placed on the esophagus. Imaging tests should be done while you're upright as well as lying down. It's also useful to have an imaging test after you've had a soft drink, so your doctor can have a good look at the stomach when it's ballooning out.

If your symptoms persist despite treatment, and all other serious diseases, such as cancer, have been completely ruled out, then you may require surgery. In this case, a procedure known as fundoplication can be done to physically increase the pressure in your lower esophagus. This is definitely a last resort that shouldn't be attempted unless all treatment options have been tried.

27. Know How to Keep GERD from Coming Back

One of the biggest problems with treating GERD is dealing with the issue of relapse. GERD has a bad habit of returning as soon as you stop your medication unless you make some dramatic lifestyle changes. The vast majority of people with GERD will reexperience their symptoms as soon as they stop their medications. This can occur within a few weeks or within six months. In fact, 85 to 90 percent of all people with GERD experience relapse. The problem with any treatment for GERD is that the medication is designed to fix things so long as you're taking it. There are no good studies that can definitely say, "When you combine drug A with drug B, you can prevent GERD from recurring." As a result, many doctors combine certain therapies based on what they've seen in their own practices; in other words, there are no "rules." Some doctors may have a lot of success combining a prokinetic drug with an H2 receptor drug, while others may find that only using omeprazole, a proton pump inhibitor, is a better way to prevent relapse. The problem with most drug studies is that they are all short term, and therefore are not useful in this instance.

The best approach to preventing relapse is to make some lifestyle changes once your initial symptoms are healed. If that doesn't work, some sort of ongoing medication may be prescribed on an intermittent basis or daily. What you take and how much you take largely depends on how well you've responded to various medications in the past and your own feelings about taking a maintenance drug. Maintenance therapy may include cisapride, an H2 receptor drug, or omeprazole, used in people who have had very severe symptoms.

28. Understand Maintenance Therapy

Unless you're prepared to make significant lifestyle changes (see Part Five), you may do well on maintenance drugs to keep your GERD symptoms at bay. If you've been prescribed medication to treat your symptoms, you'll probably be instructed to take it twice a day. Once your symptoms subside, to prevent relapse, you'll probably be prescribed a lower dosage twice a day. If you seem to suffer from symptoms at night and wake up nauseated, then taking your medication at bedtime can be done, too. If you're doing shift work and suffer from GERD only when you're working odd-hour shifts, you may be advised to take your medication as needed.

H2 receptor drugs will usually be prescribed for maintenance dosing at 800 mg at bedtime or 600 mg twice daily, while proton pump inhibitors such as omeprazole will be prescribed at 20 mg daily.

29. Ask About *H. Pylori*

Although *H. pylori* is usually a factor only in ulcer cases (see Part Two), in select cases of NUD or GERD, treating *H. pylori* has been of some benefit. It remains to be seen whether these benefits are:

- Coincidental. (John Doe stopped eating chili burgers the week he was put on antibiotics for *H. pylori* infection; it was really the chili burgers that were the problem.)
- Placebo effect. (The belief that *H. pylori* is a factor in his illness causes John Doe to get better.)
- Real. (Inflammation triggered by John Doe's *H. pylori* did, indeed, induce a motility problem.)

We just don't know which of the above is the correct answer. If your doctor does decide to treat *H. pylori* to prevent GERD relapse, see the discussion of antibiotics in the previous section.

30. Use This Table to Help You Get Diagnosed Accurately

If you can figure out whether your symptoms are "ulcer" or "not ulcer," you're on the right track to an accurate diagnosis for your upper G.I. symptoms. Table 30.1 can help steer you and your doctor in the right direction.

Table 30.1 Ulcer Symptoms

Sounds like an ulcer if:	Sounds like dysmotility if you have:	See a specialist if you are 40+ and/or suddenly notice:
you notice hunger-pang pain	heartburn that wakes you	it's hard to swallow
pain is relieved by food or antacids	reflux	weight loss
you can pinpoint pain	belching or gas	black stools
you've had an ulcer before	bloating and/or nausea and/or pain after eating	bloody saliva
you're taking aspirin or NSAIDs	pain that is hard to pinpoint	bloody vomit
there's a family history of ulcer	symptoms not relieved by antacids	chest pain
you smoke	symptoms that don't wake you	cough/asthma
you have black stools or bloody vomit		no therapy helps

PART FOUR

What to Know About Tummy Medications

31. Know What You Can Get Over the Counter

If you walk down the "stomach aisle" of any drugstore, you'll find a dizzying variety of antacids (such as Tums or Rolaids) and what are called acid-lowering drugs, acid-controlling drugs, or more to the point, acid-blocking drugs. These are the stronger drugs discussed in the previous parts, known as H2 receptor antagonists (cimetidine, famotidine, nizatidine, and ranitidine). Until recently, all H2 receptor antagonists were prescription drugs. In the United States, you can now purchase these drugs in an over-the-counter formulation, which contains less drug than the prescription version. Pepcid and Tagamet are examples of over-the-counter H2 receptor antagonists. (These drugs are still prescription only in Canada.) We often make the assumption that if something is sitting on the shelf and is sold over the counter, it can be taken every day, any time. This is not the case. And if you read the labels, the manufacturers will tell you so, themselves. Antacids are intended for mild bouts of heartburn. Unfortunately, there are many people that take them every day. If this describes your situation, see your doctor to find out what's causing your chronic condition.

32. Know the Difference Between an Antacid and an Acid Blocker

Antacids relieve heartburn (acid indigestion, sour stomach) as well as peptic ulcer disease symptoms by neutralizing stomach acid that rises up into the esophagus. There are various neutralizing agents that work on hydrochloric acid— aluminum hydroxide (Amphojel); calcium carbonate (Tums or Rolaids); magnesium (Mylanta, Maalox); or a foaming agent such as alginic acid. An interesting variant is the ever-popular Alka Seltzer. This common antacid actually contains three principal ingredients: aspirin, sodium bicarbonate, and citric acid, which, in water, forms sodium citrate and sodium acetylsalicylate. That's a lot of medication. And if you read the label, Alka Seltzer is indicated for heartburn *combined* with headache and/or aches and pains from "the overindulgence in food and drink." (Not surprisingly, Alka Seltzer is a popular hangover cure.) Foamy antacids are thought to work because the foam seems to form a barrier between the stomach and esophagus, preventing heartburn in some people.

All antacids allow you a maximum number of tablets or teaspoons per day that is fairly liberal. For example, you can take up to sixteen Tums per day. You're allowed eight tablets of Alka Seltzer per day. If you prefer a liquid form of antacid, you're allowed sixteen teaspoons of Maalox or Gaviscon per day. But you can't do this forever. All antacid labels explicitly say something such as, "Consult your physician if symptoms persist beyond two weeks." This means that your romance with antacids has to end after two weeks; if you take the maximum daily dosage every day for a period that exceeds two weeks, you could suffer from the following side effects:

- Diarrhea.

- Problems metabolizing calcium.

- A buildup of magnesium, which can aggravate or trigger kidney disease (particularly in people who have diabetes).

- Possible lead toxicity. (Currently, an environmental group is in the process of suing various antacid and calcium supplement makers, alleging that their products contain dangerous amounts of lead.)

Many antacids cannot be combined with tetracycline or anticoagulants, such as warfarin. It's always best to check with a pharmacist before you purchase any product.

Know What an Acid Blocker Is

If you have chronic heartburn or reflux, your doctor may recommend or prescribe an H2 receptor antagonist, which is different than an antacid. These medications actually inhibit your stomach from secreting acid in the first place. The four H2 receptor antagonists on the market right now are cimetidine (Tagamet), famotidine (Pepcid), nizatidine (Axid), and ranitidine (Zantac). In the United States, all these drugs are sold over the counter at lower strengths than they are available in prescription form. In Canada, these drugs remain prescription only.

H2 antagonists are always prescribed when an ulcer is diagnosed or when you suffer from gastroesophageal reflux disease (GERD). They are used mainly as a pain reliever rather than a drug that treats the underlying problem. Therefore, H2 receptor antagonists are usually recommended for short-term rather than long-term use. If you respond well to an acid-blocking drug, however, many doctors recommend that you continue to take it as maintenance therapy for a prolonged time period of anywhere from six to twelve months. That's because H2 receptor drugs are fairly safe drugs that are relatively cheap, with an easy dosing schedule of just one or two tablets per day.

If you have symptoms of dysmotility, an H2 receptor antagonist is probably not the drug for you; in this case, you need a motility, or prokinetic agent, such as cisapride, discussed further on. In fact, many people take an H2 receptor drug repeatedly without seeing their symptoms dissipate. As discussed in Item 4, this means that they probably have a motility problem, not an acid problem.

Dosages and Length of Therapy

In the early 1980s, the American Medical Association recommended that H2 receptor drugs be used for a period of two weeks to initially treat symptoms and then an additional four weeks to prevent symptoms from coming back. No doctor follows these dosing guidelines anymore. If you're not responding to H2 receptor drugs within a couple of weeks, your doctor will prescribe either a motility drug, such as cisapride, or an extremely potent acid-lowering drug known as a proton pump inhibitor, such as omeprazole (Prilosec or Losec) or lansoprazole (Prevacid), which are available only by prescription.

Dosages are all over the map; it depends on which brand you're taking. Nizatidine is taken twice a day (150 mg twice daily); prescription-strength cimetidine is taken twice a day at much higher doses (400 mg twice daily); famotidine is taken once a day (one 40 mg tablet); while ranitidine is taken twice a day (300 mg twice daily).

Drugs That Cannot Be Combined with Acid Blockers

Cimetidine cannot be combined with the following drugs:

- Anticoagulants, such as warfarin.
- Phenytoin.
- Propranolol.
- Chlordiazepoxide.
- Lidocaine.
- Diazepam.
- Theophylline.
- Nifedipine.

If you're taking any of the above medications, you can request famotidine or nizatidine. Ranitidine, specifically, cannot be combined with NSAIDs, theophylline, or oral hypoglycemic agents.

33. Understand More About Prokinetic Drugs

When your doctor says you have a motility problem or, more specifically, dysmotility, it means that your stomach's motion is impaired. In this case, the acid is in the esophagus because your digestive tract's muscles aren't coordinating well enough for the lower esophageal sphincter to work. Prokinetic drugs are prescribed for dysmotility symptoms, such as bloating and inability to finish a meal, which accompany pain and heartburn symptoms. Prokinetic drugs, as discussed in Item 24, work by restoring proper motility or motion to your digestive tract's muscles. The problem with prokinetic drugs is that many people don't take them as prescribed. When that happens, the drugs aren't dangerous in any way, but they won't work!

Until recently the most common prokinetic drug was cisapride (Propulsid; Prepulsid in Canada), but it was taken off the market. Other prokinetic drugs are metaclopramide (Maxeran) and domperidone (Motilium).

34. Understand What a Proton Pump Inhibitor Is

If antacids are "water pistols," proton pump inhibitors, such as omeprazole (Prilosec; Losec in Canada) or lansoprazole (Prevacid), are "nuclear weapons." These very potent acid-suppressing drugs are reserved for severe situations only. To take these drugs you must have:

- Severe peptic ulcer disease.
- Severe gastroesophageal reflux disease.
- Severe esophagitis.
- An esophageal ulcer.

Proton pump inhibitors are intended as a short-term therapy only. If you're taking omeprazole, for the first two weeks of therapy, you would take a 40 mg tablet four times per day, and then half that dosage for an additional two weeks. If you're prescribed lansoprazole, you would take one 15 mg tablet daily before breakfast for two to four weeks. Proton pump inhibitors are generally not recommended for longer than four weeks unless there are special circumstances. Proton pump inhibitors are also expensive drugs, compared to H2 receptor drugs; omeprazole costs roughly $75 per month compared to $10 for cimetidine. Therefore, prescribing these drugs as a maintenance therapy is inappropriate from a cost standpoint, too. Some experts describe proton pump inhibitors as "too good" a drug. In other words, once you go on the drug, it's hard to coax you off it because it does such a good job of relieving acid-related symptoms. The problem, however, is that this type of drug isn't meant to be taken for a long time.

There are many side effects to proton pump inhibitors, as well as several drug interactions.

35. Know How to Take Your Drugs to Avoid Irritating Your Stomach

Throughout this book, the issue of aspirin and nonsteroidal anti-inflammatory drugs (NSAIDs) causing pain and ulcer disease has been raised. There are several other medications that can also affect your digestive system, particularly oral medications. Many of the problems are caused by people taking medications incorrectly. For example, if you're supposed to take a drug on an empty stomach and you take it with food, or vice versa, you may be in for some nausea or vomiting. The older you get, the more vulnerable you are to digestive upset with various medications.

If you have food allergies, such as lactose or gluten intolerance, you may also have problems; lactose and gluten are often added to pills or tablets for taste and consistency.

A common problem with any pills that need to be swallowed is that they can irritate the esophagus. This is particularly the case when you're having trouble swallowing a giant "horse pill." If the pill stays in the esophagus too long, it can release its chemicals, meant for your small intestine, into the esophagus and irritate the lining. This can cause ulcers, bleeding, tearing, or inflammation. As a result, you'll experience pain when you swallow liquid or solid food. You may also literally feel the tablet lodged in your throat (eat a hearty crust of bread to get it down, in this case). You may also feel a dull ache in your chest or shoulder (that means the pain has radiated into your shoulder; the pill isn't in your shoulder, however) after you take the irritating medication. People especially susceptible to these problems include anyone with:

- Esophagitis.
- Scleroderma (hardening of the skin).
- Achalasia (irregular muscle activity of the esophagus).
- A history of strokes.

How to Swallow Pills

Experts recommend you swallow tablets in a standing position. If you're bedridden or confined to a chair, sitting upright is best. Before taking a pill, swallow some liquid to lubricate your throat first, then take your pill with a full glass of liquid. After you swallow the pill, wait at least fifteen minutes before you lie down to make sure that the pill is safely past your esophagus.

Certain drugs can cause reflux, even if you've done everything in your power to swallow correctly. These drugs range from calcium channel blockers to oral contraceptives. In this case, all you can do is wait for the reflux episode to pass and avoid other reflux triggers, discussed in Item 3.

36. Know the Drugs That Can Irritate Your Stomach

If you're taking a nonsteroidal anti-inflammatory drug (NSAID), such as ibuprofen or naproxyn, the lining of your stomach can become irritated. In fact, in the absence of the bacterial infection *H. pylori*, NSAIDs and aspirin use are the most common cause of ulcers.

Like *H. pylori*, NSAIDs can weaken the stomach lining's ability to resist its own acid. The older you are, the more at risk you are for NSAID-induced stomach irritation because you're more likely to be taking NSAIDs as pain relievers for arthritic conditions. Requesting coated tablets, avoiding alcohol, and taking your pills with milk or water can be somewhat helpful, but not a guarantee.

Anticholinergics, antidepressants, and drugs used to treat Parkinson's disease are notorious for causing motility problems. In this case, there is no magic technique you can employ before, during, or after taking your drug that can prevent dysmotility. The only remedy is switching to a different medication, or taking a motility agent such as cisapride along with the culprit medication.

37. Know the Drugs That Cause Bowel Problems

The most common side effects of any medications are constipation or diarrhea. Although this is a lower G.I. story, it can complicate the effectiveness of any and all drugs you're taking, including drugs for upper G.I. problems. Constipation is caused by any drug that affects the nerves and muscle activity in your colon. When this happens, your stools are slow to come, and hard when they do come! Anti-hypertensives, anticholinergics, cholestyramine, iron, and aluminum-containing antacids are the most common offenders.

As for diarrhea, antibiotics will usually cause this because they kill off bacteria that normally live in your colon, which are there for good reason. Without this friendly bowel bacteria, the overgrowth of another bacteria, called *Clostridium difficile (C. difficile)*, will take place. *C. difficile* is actually responsible for colitis (inflammation of the colon). In response, the colon secretes excess water, which is what makes the stools runny, creating consistencies ranging from stews to juice. If you're taking a lot of antibiotics, you may want to request alternatives to ampicillin, clindamycin, and the cephalosporins class of drugs; these are the ones that cause the most problems. How do you treat antibiotic-related diarrhea or colitis? The punchline is—with another antibiotic (one that kills off *C. difficile*).

Some drugs cause diarrhea simply because they "make water" in your colon. In this case, you do not have any inflammation, just too much fluid in the colon. Drugs known to do this are colchicine and magnesium-containing antacids. Finally, laxatives will often cause diarrhea because people tend to overuse them or abuse them. In this case, permanent damage to the nerves and muscles of the colon will cause chronic diarrhea.

Occasionally, the drug misoprostol is prescribed in cases where NSAIDs and/or aspirin have caused an ulcer. More commonly, however, misoprostol is prescribed "off label" as a drug to induce abortion, as well as to prevent hemorrhaging after childbirth. It would never be prescribed to you during pregnancy, but if you think you might be pregnant, make sure you disclose this to your doctor before filling a prescription for misoprostol.

38. Know About a Dozen Irritating Drugs

The following common drugs can irritate your stomach. By asking your doctor for alternatives to these medications, you may be able to alleviate upper G.I. symptoms:

1. Acetaminophen: (Tylenol, Panadol, and Datril).

2. Antibiotics: penicillin (Amoxil, Amcil, and Augmentin), clindamycin, cephalosporins (Keflex and Ceclor), tetracyclines (Minocin, Sumycin, and Vibramycin), quinolones (Cipro), and sulfa drugs (Bactrim).

3. Anticholinergics: propantheline (Pro-Banthine), dicyclomine (Bentyl), amitriptyline (Elavil and Endep), nortriptyline (Aventyl and Pamelor), levodopa (Dopar), and carbidopa and levodopa combination (Sinemet).

4. Anticonvulsants: phenytoin (Dilantin) and valproic acid (Dalpro).

5. Antihypertensives: warfarin.

6. Calcium channel blockers: diltiazem (Cardizem), nifedipine (Procardia), and verapamil (Isoptin).

7. Chlorpromazine: Thorazine and Ormazine.

8. Colchicine.

9. Nitrates: isosorbide dinitrate (Iso-Bid and Isonate) and nitroglycerin (Nitro-Bid and Nitrocap).

10. Nonsteroidal anti-inflammatory drugs (NSAIDs): aspirin (Bayer and Bufferin), ibuprofen (Advil, Nuprin, and Motrin), tolmetin (Tolectin), naproxen (Naprosyn), and piroxicam (Feldene).
11. Quinidine: Quinalan and Quiniglute.
12. Theophylline: TheoDur, Theophyl, and Bronkodyl.

39. Be Informed About All Your Drugs

You are entitled to full information about all the drugs you take. Chances are, most of the drugs you take are powerful. Without exception, most drugs currently being prescribed have a long list of possible side effects. So the first question you must always ask before you take any prescribed drug is: What are the side effects? Many doctors have ethical problems with disclosing all potential side effects of the drugs they prescribe because you might "freak out" if you knew about all of them. It's akin to an airline passenger reading about all the things that could go wrong with a plane before he flies. Do you really want to know? I can't answer that question for you; only you can. (You know your information threshold better than I do.) But in general, when you ask your doctor about side effects, she'll disclose the most common ones. The drug's manufacturer will also have patient information available toll free or on an advertised website. If you insist on being told about rare and unlikely side effects, your doctor or pharmacist cannot legally withhold this information from you. If he does, and you're willing to risk unnecessary anxiety in exchange for probably way too much information, you can always look up the drug in the *Physician's Desk Reference* (PDR), available in your local library. (Chances are you won't understand most of what you read because it's so technical; but if you take a photocopy to your doctor or pharmacist, he can explain what it says, and probably alleviate some fears.) It's also crucial to ask how diet, certain activities, and exercise can affect your medications. The following questions should always be asked about prescription drugs:

- How do these drugs affect my fertility, a pregnancy, or breastfeeding? If they should not be taken during pregnancy or breastfeeding, ask for safe alternatives. For example, many drugs pass through the placenta, or can be excreted through breast milk.

- What are the alternative therapies? Are there less severe therapies (for example, herbs)?

- What other therapies will be combined with this drug? Many drugs are prescribed in combination.

- How long does it take before I begin to feel better? This asks about the drug's efficacy or effectiveness.

- What drugs or substances should not be combined with this drug? This asks about contraindications to the drug. For example, can you have wine? Cough medicine? Caffeine?

- How does this drug interact with other prescription drugs or over-the-counter medications I'm taking? Whether you're taking aspirin or drinking herbal tea, find out.

- How does my medical history affect the potency or toxicity of this drug? Have you had any major surgeries? Do you have diabetes? Do you have a history of seizures? Problems can turn up if you don't ask this question.

- How long does it stay in my system after I go off? Even when you're off a drug, it could have a long half-life and still interact with other drugs you may take.

- Can I stop the medication as soon as I feel better? Great question. Usually the answer is "no" with prescription medications, as they are not meant to be taken on an as-needed basis.

- How often do I have to take the drug and when is the best time to take it? Some drugs need to be taken three times a day, some once a day. Some drugs need to be taken at bedtime, some with meals. Make sure you have all this information. It could make a difference between good and bad side effects, potency, or how long the drug stays in your system.

- What if I miss a dose? Sometimes the answer is to double up; other times you're told to skip it and carry on. This entirely depends on the medication, manufacturer, and dosage.

Drug Studies

Obviously what's needed in drug treatment for a variety of ailments are effective drugs with few side effects. Therefore, the impetus to create new and improved drugs is always there. But that also means it's necessary to test the drugs on real people to see if they work better than the standard therapy. It's therefore not at all unusual for you to be approached to participate in a drug study (also known as a clinical trial). Some studies are more ethical than others, however. It's perfectly reasonable, for example, to test the standard therapy against a new therapy. That's the only way to see whether the new therapy will be better, which is the only method of raising the standard for future patients.

But when you're suffering from an illness for which there is good, safe, and effective medication, it's not reasonable to ask you to participate in what is known as a placebo-controlled trial. Here, some people receive standard therapy in the form of real medication, while other people receive "dummy therapy" in the form of a fake pill that is made of a sugar solution. The purpose of a placebo-controlled trial is to test whether the real medication is really "better than nothing." In order to do this, what's known as double-blinded studies are done, in which people are told that they may receive either a fake pill or real pill. You won't know what you're given until the trial is over. Often, it becomes obvious who's getting the real pills, and in these cases, the trials are stopped (or at least, ought to be stopped). But many studies have found that the placebo effect (the belief that the medication is working) can often be enough to cure an ailment or illness, proving that sometimes the drug really isn't better than nothing. With most severe illnesses, we already know that without medication, a lot of people suffer needlessly. So when a good, effective, standard therapy exists to relieve your suffering, it is considered by many bioethicists to be unethical to give you nothing. That doesn't mean that placebo-controlled trials don't go on; it simply means that you ought to question whether it's fair to you to participate.

Informed Consent and Medication

Legally, if you are being subjected to a treatment without your consent, it constitutes battery. If you are treated without adequate informed consent, it constitutes negligence.

This applies to consenting to medication, drug trials, or any other form of therapy. So to make sure you are being adequately informed, the following three things must occur:

1. Disclosure. Have you been provided with relevant and comprehensive information by your health care provider? According to medical ethicists, disclosure means that a description of the treatment, its expected result, information about relevant alternative options and their expected benefits and relevant risks, and an explanation of the consequences of declining or delaying treatment must be provided. You should also be given an opportunity to ask questions, and your health care providers should be available to answer them.

2. Capacity to consent. Do you understand information relevant to a treatment decision, and do you appreciate the reasonably foreseeable consequences of a decision or lack of one? Do you understand what's being disclosed, and can you decide on your treatment based on this information?

3. Voluntariness. Are you being allowed to make your health care choice free of any undue influences? Is information being distorted or omitted? Is someone (even a family member) forcing you, manipulating you, or coercing you into a decision that goes against your instincts?

If you use the above as a checklist, you'll be able to make as informed a choice as anyone can expect from a layperson.

40. Know the Right Drug Routes

When you're diagnosed with chronic heartburn/reflux, use the following steps as a guide for which drugs should be prescribed at what time.

- Start by modifying your diet and lifestyle habits with or without over-the-counter antacids.

- If you don't find relief, your doctor can prescribe a prokinetic agent (cisapride) or an H2 receptor antagonist (cimetidine, famotidine, nizatidine, or ranitidine).

- If you're still not finding relief, your doctor can prescribe a proton pump inhibitor (omeprazole, lansoprozole) or rule out a more serious condition with tests.

PART FIVE

Preventing Upper G.I. Disorders

41. Understand Why You Should Quit Smoking

Smoking isn't just hard on the lungs and heart—it's hard on the gut. So if you're suffering from upper G.I. problems and you smoke, by quitting smoking, you may be able to make your symptoms vanish.

Aside from that, roughly half a million North Americans die of smoking-related illnesses each year. That's 20 percent of all deaths from all causes. We already know that smoking causes lung cancer. But did you know that smokers are also twice as likely to develop heart disease? Lesser known long-term effects of smoking include lowering of HDL, or "good" cholesterol, and damage to the lining of blood vessel walls, which paves the way for arterial plaque formation. In addition to increasing the risk of lung cancer and heart disease, smoking can lead to stroke, peripheral vascular disease, and a host of other cancers.

Like a good cigar or a pipe once in a while? Forget it— cigars are bad for the gut, too. When you smoke a cigar, you're getting filler, binder, and wrapper, which are made of air-cured and fermented tobaccos. Like cigarette tobacco, lit cigars emit over four thousand chemicals, of which forty-three are known to cause cancer—many of them G.I. cancers.

Cigar smokers have higher death rates than nonsmokers for most smoking-related diseases, although not nearly as high as cigarette smokers. When the nicotine is absorbed through the mouth, however, cigar/pipe smokers, as well as anyone using chewing tobacco or snuff, are at higher risk of laryngeal, oral, and esophageal cancer. Cigar/pipe smokers also have higher death rates than nonsmokers from chronic obstructive lung disease as well as lung cancer.

So whether it's cigars, cigarettes, or even chewing tobacco (snuff), take a look at some of the things you'll gain by quitting smoking:

- Improved digestion and sense of taste.
- Decreased risk of heart disease.
- Decreased risk of cancer (that includes of the lung, esophagus, mouth, throat, pancreas, kidney, bladder, and cervix).
- Lower heart rate and blood pressure.
- Decreased risk of lung disease (bronchitis, emphysema).
- Relaxation of blood vessels.
- Better teeth.
- Fewer wrinkles.

Take a Look at What You're Inhaling

In 1989, the U.S. Surgeon General released a report listing forty-three carcinogenic agents found in tobacco smoke. The IARC (International Agency for Research on Cancer) classified them as follows:

Group 1A—Carcinogenic to Humans

Tobacco smoke

Tobacco products, smokeless

4-Aminobiphenyl

Benzene

Cadmium

Chromium

2-Naphthylamine

Nickel

Polonium

Polonium-210 (radon)

Vinyl chloride

Group 2A—Probably Carcinogenic to Humans

Acrylonitrile

Benzo[a]anthracene

Benzo[a]pyrene

1,3-Butadiene

Dibenz[a,h]anthracene

Formaldehyde

N-Nitrosodiethylamine

N-Nitrosodimethlamine

Group 2B — Possibly Carcinogenic to Humans

Acetaldehyde
Benzo[b]fluoranthene
Benzo[j]fluoranthene
Benzo[k]fluoranthene
Dibenz[a,h]acridine
Dibenz[a,j]acridine
7H-Dibenz[c,g]carbazole
Dibenzo[a,l]pyrene
1,1-Dimethylhydrazine
Hydrazine
Indeno-2,3-c[d]pyrene
Lead
5-Methylchrysene
4-(Methylnitrosamine)-2-(3-pyridyl)-1-butanene (NNK)
2-Nitropropane
N-Nitrosodiethanolamine
N-Nitrosomethylethylamine
N-Nitrosomorpholine
N-Nitrosopyrrolidine
Quinoline
Ortho-Toluidine
Urethane (ethyl carbamate)

Group 3 — Unclassified as to Carcinogenicity to Humans (Limited Evidence)

Chrysene
Crotonaldehyde
N-Nitrosoanabasine (NAB)
N-Nitrosoanatabine (NAT)

42. Understand How to Quit Smoking

Not everyone can quit smoking "cold turkey," although it's a strategy that many have used successfully. (Some cold turkey quitters report that keeping one package of cigarettes within reach lessens anxiety.) The symptoms of nicotine withdrawal begin within a few hours and peak at twenty-four to forty-eight hours after quitting. You may experience anxiety, irritability, hostility, restlessness, insomnia, and anger. For these reasons, many smokers turn to smoking cessation programs, which can include some of the following:

- Behavioral counseling. Behavioral counseling, either group or individual, can raise the rate of abstinence from 20 to 25 percent. This approach to smoking cessation aims to change the mental processes of smoking, reinforce the benefits of nonsmoking, and teach skills to help the smoker avoid the urge to smoke.

- Nicotine gum. Nicotine gum (Nicorette) is now available over the counter. It works as an aid to help you quit smoking by reducing nicotine cravings and withdrawal symptoms. Nicotine gum helps you wean yourself from nicotine by allowing you to gradually decrease the dosage until you stop using it altogether, a process that usually takes about twelve weeks. The only disadvantage to this method is that it caters to the oral and addictive aspects of smoking (rewarding the urge to smoke with a dose of nicotine).

- Nicotine patch. Transdermal nicotine, or the patch (Habitrol, Nicoderm, Nicotrol), doubles abstinence rates in former smokers. Most brands are now available over the counter. Each morning, a new patch is applied to a different area of dry, clean, hairless skin and left on for the day. Some patches are designed to be worn a full twenty-four hours. The constant supply of nicotine to the bloodstream sometimes causes very vivid or disturbing dreams, however. You can also expect to feel a mild itching, burning, or tingling at the site of the patch when it is first applied. The nicotine patch works best when it is worn for at least seven to twelve weeks, with a gradual decrease in strength (nicotine). Many smokers find it effective because it allows them to tackle the psychological addiction to smoking before they are forced to deal with physical symptoms of withdrawal.

- Nicotine inhaler. The nicotine inhaler (Nicotrol Inhaler) delivers nicotine orally via inhalation from a plastic tube. Its success rate is about 28 percent, similar to that of nicotine gum. It's available by prescription only in the United States and has yet to make its debut in Canada. Like nicotine gum, the inhaler mimics smoking behavior by responding to each craving or urge to smoke, a feature with both advantages and disadvantages to the smoker who wants to get over the physical symptoms of withdrawal. The nicotine inhaler should be used for a period of twelve weeks.

- Nicotine nasal spray. Like nicotine gum and the nicotine patch, the nasal spray reduces craving and withdrawal symptoms, allowing smokers to cut back gradually. One squirt delivers about 1 mg nicotine. In three clinical trials involving 730 patients, 31 to 35 percent were not smoking at six months. This compares to an average of 12 to 15 percent of smokers who were able to quit unaided. The nasal spray has a couple of advantages over the gum and the patch: nicotine is rapidly absorbed across the nasal membranes, providing a kick that is more like the real thing; and the prompt onset of action plus a flexible dosing schedule benefits heavier smokers. Because the nicotine reaches the bloodstream so quickly, nasal sprays do have a greater potential for addiction than the slower acting gum and patch. Nasal sprays are not yet available for use in Canada.

- Alternative therapies. Hypnosis, meditation, and acupuncture have helped some smokers quit. In the case of hypnosis and meditation, sessions may be private or part of a group smoking cessation program.

Drugs That Help You Quit

The drug bupropion (Zyban) is now available, and is an option for people who have been unsuccessful using nicotine replacement. Formerly prescribed as an antidepressant, bupropion was discovered by accident; researchers knew that smokers who had quit were often depressed, and so they began experimenting with the drug as a means to fight depression, not addiction. Bupropion reduces the withdrawal symptoms associated with smoking cessation and can be used in conjunction with nicotine replacement therapy. Researchers suspect that bupropion works directly in the brain to disrupt the addictive power of nicotine by affecting the same chemical neurotransmitters (or messengers) in the brain, such as dopamine, that nicotine does.

The pleasurable aspect of addictive drugs, such as nicotine and cocaine, is triggered by the release of dopamine.

Smoking floods the brain with dopamine. *The New England Journal of Medicine* published the results of a study of more than six hundred smokers taking bupropion. At the end of treatment, 44 percent of those who took the highest dose of the drug (300 mg) were not smoking, compared to 19 percent of the group who took a placebo. By the end of one year, 23 percent of the 300 mg group and 12 percent of the placebo group were still smoke free. Using Zyban with nicotine replacement therapy seems to improve the quit rate a bit further. Four-week quit rates from the study were 23 percent for placebo, 36 percent for the patch, 49 percent for Zyban, and 58 percent for Zyban and the patch combined.

43. Cut the Fat

When people who suffer from upper G.I. problems lose weight and cut down on fat, they feel better, and often their G.I. symptoms disappear. But it's hard to cut down on fat unless you really understand what fat is! Fat is technically known as fatty acids, which are crucial nutrients for our cells. We cannot live without fatty acids, or fat. If you looked at each fat molecule carefully, you'd find three different kinds of fatty acids on it: saturated (solid), monounsaturated (less solid, with the exception of olive and peanut oils), and polyunsaturated (liquid) fatty acids. When you see the term *unsaturated fat*, this refers to either monounsaturated or polyunsaturated fats.

These three fatty acids combine with glycerol to make what's chemically known as triglycerides. Each fat molecule is a link in a chain made up of glycerol, carbon atoms, and hydrogen atoms. The more hydrogen atoms that are on that chain, the more saturated or solid the fat. The liver breaks down fat molecules by secreting bile (stored in the gall-bladder) — its sole function. The liver also makes cholesterol. Too much saturated fat may cause your liver to overproduce cholesterol, while the triglycerides in your bloodstream will rise, perpetuating the problem.

Fat is therefore a good thing — in moderation. But like all good things, most of us want too much of it. Excess dietary fat is by far the most damaging element in the Western diet. A gram of fat contains twice the calories as the same amount of protein or carbohydrate. Decreasing the fat in your diet and replacing it with more grain products, vegetables, and fruit is the best way to lower your risk of colon cancer and cardiovascular diseases. Fat in the diet comes from meats, dairy products, and vegetable oils. Other sources of fat include coconuts (60 percent fat), peanuts (78 percent fat), and avocados (82 percent fat). There are different kinds of fatty acids in these sources of fats: saturated, monounsaturated, and polyunsaturated (which, again, is what is meant by unsaturated fat). Additionally, there is a fourth kind of fat in our diets: transfatty acids. These are factory-made fats that are found in margarines, for example.

To cut through all this big, fat jargon, you can boil down fat into two categories: harmful fats and helpful fats (which the popular press often defines as good fats and bad fats).

Harmful Fats

The following are harmful fats because they can increase your risk of cardiovascular problems, as well as many cancers, including colon and breast cancers. These are fats that are fine in moderation, but harmful in excess (and harmless if not eaten at all):

- Saturated fats. These are solid at room temperature and stimulate cholesterol production in your body. In fact, the way that saturated fat looks prior to ingesting it is the way it will look when it lines your arteries. Foods high in saturated fat include processed meat, fatty meat, lard, butter, margarine, solid vegetable shortening, chocolate, and tropical oils (coconut oil is more than 90 percent saturated). Saturated fat should be consumed only in very small amounts.

- Transfatty acids. These are factory-made fats that behave just like saturated fat in your body.

Helpful Fats

These are fats that are beneficial to your health and actually protect against certain health problems, such as cardiovascular disease. You are encouraged to use these fats more, rather than less frequently, in your diet. In fact, nutritionists suggest that you substitute harmful fats with these:

- Unsaturated fat. This is partially solid or liquid at room temperature. The more liquid the fat, the more polyunsaturated it is, which, in fact, lowers your cholesterol levels. This group of fats includes monounsaturated fats and polyunsaturated fats. Sources of unsaturated fats include vegetable oils (canola, safflower, sunflower, corn) and seeds and nuts. Unsaturated fats come from plants, with the exception of tropical oils, such as coconut.

- Fish fats (omega-3 oils). The fats naturally present in fish that swim in cold waters, known as omega-3 fatty acids or fish oils, are all polyunsaturated. Again, poly-unsaturated fats are good for you: they lower choles-terol levels, are crucial for brain tissue, and protect against heart disease. Look for cold-water fish such as mackerel, albacore tuna, salmon, and sardines.

About Carbs

Fat is not the only thing that can make you fat; what about carbohydrates? You see, a diet high in carbohydrates can also make you fat. That's because carbohydrates—meaning starchy stuff, such as rice, pasta, breads, or potatoes—can be stored as fat when eaten in excess.

Carbohydrates can be simple or complex. Simple car-bohydrates are found in any food that has natural sugar (honey, fruits, juices, vegetables, milk) and anything that contains table sugar. Complex carbohydrates are more sophisticated foods that are made up of larger molecules, such as grain foods, starches, and foods high in fiber.

Normally, all carbs convert into glucose when you eat them. Glucose is the technical term for simplest sugar. All your energy comes from glucose in your blood—also known as blood glucose or blood sugar—your body fuel. When your blood sugar is used up, you feel weak, tired, and hun-gry. But what happens when you eat more carbohydrates than your body can use? Your body will store those extra carbs as fat. What we also know is that the rate at which glucose is absorbed by your body from carbohydrates is affected by other parts of your meal, such as protein, fiber, and fat. If you're eating only carbohydrates and no protein or fat, for example, they will convert into glucose more quickly—to the point where you may feel mood swings as your blood sugar rises and dips. Nutrition experts advise

that you should consume roughly 50 to 55 percent carbohydrates, 15 to 20 percent protein, and less than 30 percent
fat daily for a healthy diet.

By making the following swaps from Table 43.1, you can
significantly lower your dietary fat:

Table 43.1

Swap	For
Hamburgers	Veggie burgers or chicken-breast sandwiches
Ground beef	Ground turkey or tofu (soybean curd)
Butter	Yogurt, hummus, or reduced-fat margarine
Homogenized milk	Skim milk or 1% milk
Soft drinks	Club soda or water

Here are some other ways to trim the fat:

- Whenever you refrigerate animal fat (in soups,
  stews, or curry dishes), skim the fat from the top
  before reheating and serving. A gravy skimmer will
  also help skim fats; the spout pours from the bottom
  while the oils and fats coagulate on top.

- Powdered nonfat milk is in vogue again; it's high in
  calcium, low in fat. Substitute it for any recipe calling for milk or cream.

- Dig out fruit recipes for dessert. Sorbet with low-fat
  yogurt topping, for example, can be elegant.
  Remember that fruit must be planned for in a
  diabetes meal plan.

- Season low-fat foods well. That way, you won't miss
  the flavor that fat adds.

- Low-fat protein comes from vegetable sources (whole grains and bean products); high-fat protein comes from animal sources.

If you're preparing meat:

- Broil, grill, or boil meat instead of frying, baking, or roasting it. (If you drain fat and cook in water, baking/roasting should be fine.)

- Trim off all visible fat from meat before and after cooking.

- Adding flour, bread crumbs, or other coatings to lean meat adds calories, and hence fat.

- Try substituting low-fat turkey meat for red meat.

Learning to read the fat content in milk is also a good way to cut down:

- Whole milk is made up of 48 percent calories from fat.

- 2% milk gets 37 percent of its calories from fat.

- 1% milk gets 26 percent of its calories from fat.

- Skim milk is completely fat free.

- Cheese gets 50 percent of its calories from fat, unless it's skim milk cheese.

- Butter gets 95 percent of its calories from fat.

- Yogurt gets 15 percent of its calories from fat.

About Sugar

Sugars are found naturally in many foods you eat. The simplest form of sugar is glucose, which is what blood sugar, also called blood glucose is—your basic body fuel. You can buy pure glucose at any drugstore in the form of dextrose tablets. Dextrose is just edible glucose. For example, when you see people having "sugar water" fed to them intravenously, dextrose is the sugar in that water. When you see dextrose on a candy-bar label, it means that the candy-bar manufacturer used edible glucose in the recipe.

Glucose is the baseline ingredient of all naturally occurring sugars, which include:

- Sucrose: table or white sugar, naturally found in sugar cane and sugar beets.
- Fructose: the natural sugar in fruits and vegetables.
- Lactose: the natural sugar in all milk products.
- Maltose: the natural sugar in grains (flours and cereals).

When you ingest a natural sugar of any kind, you're actually ingesting one part glucose and one or two parts of another naturally occurring sugar. For example, sucrose is biochemically constructed from one part glucose and one part fructose. So, from glucose it came, and unto glucose it shall return—once it hits your digestive system. The same is true for all naturally occurring sugars, with the exception of lactose. As it happens, lactose breaks down into glucose and an odd duck simple sugar, galactose (which I used to think was something in our solar system until I became a health writer). Just think of lactose as the Milky Way and you'll probably remember.

Simple sugars can get pretty complicated when you discuss their molecular structures. For example, simple sugars can be classified as monosaccharides (single sugars) or disaccharides (double sugars). But unless you're writing a chemistry exam on sugars, you don't need to know this confusing stuff: You just need to know that all naturally occurring sugars wind up as glucose once you eat them. Glucose is carried to your cells through the bloodstream and is used as body fuel or energy.

How long does it take for one of the above sugars to return to glucose? Well, it greatly depends on the amount of fiber in your food, how much protein you've eaten, and how much fat accompanies the sugar in your meal. As stated elsewhere, if you have enough energy or fuel, once that sugar becomes glucose, it can be stored as fat. And that's how—and why—sugar can make you fat.

What you have to watch out for is added sugar; these are sugars that manufacturers add to foods during processing or packaging. Foods containing fruit juice concentrates, invert sugar, regular corn syrup, honey, molasses, hydrolyzed lactose syrup, or high-fructose corn syrup (made out of highly concentrated fructose through the hydrolysis of starch), all have added sugars. Many people don't realize, however, that pure, unsweetened fruit juice is still a potent source of sugar, even when it contains no added sugar. Extra lactose (naturally occurring sugar in milk products), dextrose (edible glucose), and maltose (naturally occurring sugar in grains) are also in many of your foods. In other words, products may have naturally occurring sugars anyway, and then more sugar is thrown in to enhance consistency, taste, and so on. The best way to know how much sugar is in a product is to look at the nutritional label for carbohydrates.

Sweeteners

Here's what you need to know about sweeteners if you're trying to cut down on fat. Although artificial sweeteners do not contain sugar (for diabetics, this means they will not affect blood sugar levels), they may contain a tiny amount of calories. It depends on whether the sweetener is classified as nutritive or nonnutritive.

Nutritive sweeteners have calories or contain natural sugar. White or brown table sugar, molasses, honey, and syrup are all considered nutritive sweeteners. Sugar alcohols are also nutritive sweeteners because they are made from fruits or produced commercially from dextrose. Sorbitol, mannitol, xylitol, and maltitol are all sugar alcohols. Sugar alcohols contain only four calories per gram, like ordinary sugar, and will affect your blood sugar levels like ordinary sugar. It all depends on how much is consumed and the degree of absorption from your digestive tract.

Nonnutritive sweeteners are sugar substitutes or artificial sweeteners; they do not have any calories and will not affect your blood sugar levels. Examples of nonnutritive sweeteners are saccharin, cyclamate, aspartame, sucralose, and acesulflame potassium.

In the 1980s, aspartame was invented, which is sold as NutraSweet. It was considered a nutritive sweetener because it was derived from natural sources (two amino acids, aspartic acid, and phenylalanine), which means that aspartame is digested and metabolized the same way as any other protein food. For every gram of aspartame, there are four calories. But since aspartame is 200 times sweeter than sugar, you don't need very much of it to achieve the desired sweetness. In at least ninety countries, aspartame is found in more than one hundred fifty product categories, including breakfast cereals, beverages, desserts, candy and gum, syrups, salad dressings, and various snack foods. Here's where it gets confusing: Aspartame is also available as a tabletop sweetener under the brand name Equal, and most recently, Prosweet. An interesting point about aspartame is that it's not recommended for baking or any other recipe where heat is required. The two amino acids in it separate with heat and the product loses its sweetness. That's not to say it's harmful if heated, but your recipe won't turn out correctly.

For the moment, aspartame is considered safe for everybody, including people with diabetes, pregnant women, and children. The only people who are cautioned against consuming it are those with a rare hereditary disease known as phenylketonuria (PKU) because aspartame contains phenylalanine, which people with PKU cannot tolerate.

Another common tabletop sweetener is sucralose, sold as Splenda. Splenda is a white crystalline powder, actually made from sugar itself. It's 600 times sweeter than table sugar but it is not broken down in your digestive system, so it has no calories at all. Splenda can also be used in hot or cold foods, and is found in hot and cold beverages, frozen foods, baked goods, and other packaged foods.

In the United States, you can still purchase cyclamate, a nonnutritive sweetener sold under the brand name Sucaryl or Sugar Twin. Cyclamate is also the sweetener used in many weight control products and is thirty times sweeter than table sugar, with no aftertaste. Cyclamate is fine for hot or cold foods. In Canada, however, you can only find cyclamate as Sugar Twin or as a sugar substitute in medication.

Sugar Alcohols

Not to be confused with alcoholic beverages, sugar alcohols are nutritive sweeteners, like regular sugar. These are found naturally in fruits or manufactured from carbohydrates. Sorbitol, mannitol, xylitol, maltitol, maltitol syrup, lactitol, isomalt, and hydrogenated starch hydrolysates are all sugar alcohols. In your body, these types of sugars are absorbed lower down in the digestive tract and will cause gastrointestinal symptoms if you use too much. Because sugar alcohols are absorbed slowly, they were once touted as ideal for people with diabetes, but since they are a carbohydrate, they still increase your blood sugar—just like regular sugar. Now that artificial sweeteners are on the market in abundance, the only real advantage of sugar alcohols is that they don't cause cavities. The bacteria in your mouth doesn't like sugar alcohols as much as real sugar.

According to the Food and Drug Administration (FDA), even foods that contain sugar alcohols can be labeled "sugar free." Sugar alcohol products can also be labeled "does not promote tooth decay," which is often confused with "low calorie."

Reading Labels

Since 1993, food labels have been adhering to strict guidelines set out by the FDA and the U.S. Department of Agriculture's (USDA) Food Safety and Inspection Service (FSIS). All labels list "Nutrition Facts" on the side or back of the package. The "Percent Daily Values" column tells you how high or low that food is in various nutrients, such as fat, saturated fat, and cholesterol. A number of 5 or less is low—good news if the product shows <5 for fat, saturated fat, and cholesterol, bad news if the product is <5 for fiber. Serving sizes are also confusing. Foods that are similar are given the same type of serving size defined by the FDA. That means that five cereals that all weigh X grams per cup will share the same serving sizes.

Calories (how much energy) and calories from fat (how much fat) are also listed per serving of food. Total carbohydrates, dietary fiber, sugars, other carbohydrates (which means starches), total fat, saturated fat, cholesterol, sodium, potassium, and vitamins and minerals are given in Percent Daily Values, based on the 2,000-calorie diet recommended by the U.S. government. (In Canada, Recommended Nutrient Intake (RNI) is used for vitamins and minerals, while ingredients on labels are listed according to weight, with the "most" listed first.)

But that's not where the confusion ends—or even begins! You have to wade through the various claims and understand what they mean. For example, anything that is "X free" (as in sugar free, saturated-fat free, cholesterol free, sodium free, calorie free, and so on) means that the product indeed has "no X" or that "X" is so tiny, it is dietarily insignificant. This is not the same thing as a label that says "95 percent fat free." In this case, the product contains relatively small amounts of fat but still has fat. This claim is based on 100 grams of the product. For example, if a snack food contains 2.5 grams of fat per 50 grams, it can be said to be 95 percent fat free.

A label that screams "low in saturated fat" or "low in calories" doesn't mean the food is fat free or calorie free. It means that you can eat a large amount of that food without exceeding the Daily Value for that food. In potato-chip country, that could mean you can eat twelve potato chips instead of six. So if you eat the whole bag of low-fat chips, you're still eating a lot of fat. Be sure to check serving sizes.

"Cholesterol free" or "low cholesterol" means that the product doesn't have any, or much, animal fat (hence, cholesterol). This doesn't mean low fat. Pure vegetable oil doesn't come from animals but is pure fat!

And then there are the comparison claims, such as "fewer," "reduced," "less," "more," or my favorite, "light" (or worse, "lite"!). These words appear on foods that have been nutritionally altered from a previous version or competitor's version. For example, Regular Brand X Potato Chips may have much more fat than Lite Brand X Potato Chips "with less fat than Regular Brand X." That doesn't mean that Lite Brand X is fat free, or even low in fat. It just means it's lower in fat than Regular Brand X.

On the flip side, Brand Y cereal may have a trace amount of calcium, while Brand X—"now with more calcium"—may still have a small amount of calcium, but 10 percent more than Brand Y. (In other words, you may still need to eat one hundred bowls of Brand Y before you get the daily requirement for calcium!)

To be light, or "lite," a product has to contain either one-third fewer calories or half the fat of the regular product. Or, a low-calorie or low-fat food might contain 50 percent less sodium. Something that is "light in sodium" means it has at least 50 percent less sodium than the regular product, such as canned soup. (But if you're buying hair color that reads "light brown," it is a descriptive word, not referring to an ingredient!)

When a label says "sugar free," the food contains less than 0.5 grams of sugars per serving, while a "reduced-sugar" food contains at least 25 percent less sugar per serving than the regular product. If the label also states that the product is not a reduced-calorie or low-calorie food, or it is not for weight control, it's got enough sugar to make you think twice.

But sugar free in the language of labels simply means sucrose free. That doesn't mean the product is carbohydrate free, as in dextrose free, lactose free, glucose free, or fructose free. Check the labels for all things ending in "ose" to find out the sugar content; you're not just looking for sucrose. Watch out for "no added sugar," "without added sugar," or "no sugar added." This simply means, "We didn't put the sugar in, God did." Again, reading the number of carbohydrates on the nutrition information label is the most accurate way to know the amount of sugar in the product.

Biological Causes of Obesity

Eating too much high-fat or high-calorie food while remaining sedentary is certainly one biological cause of obesity. Furthermore, a woman's metabolism slows down by 25 percent after menopause, which means that unless she either decreases her calories by 25 percent or increases her activity level by 25 percent to compensate, she will probably gain weight. There are also other hormonal problems that can contribute to obesity, such as an underactive thyroid gland (called hypothyroidism), which is very common in women over fifty.

Since diet and lifestyle changes are so difficult, there is an interest in finding genetic causes for obesity. That would mean that obesity is beyond our control—and something we've inherited, which would probably be comforting for many people. Now that we are amidst the Human Genome Project, a project that intends to map every gene in the human body, efforts are underway to find the "obesity gene" or "fat gene." But few scientists believe that obesity is simply genetic. In other words, there are so many environmental and social factors that can trip the obesity switch, finding a specific gene for obesity is about as worthwhile as finding the "anger gene" or "crime gene."

An important theory about why we get fat involves insulin resistance. It's believed that when the body produces too much insulin, we will eat more to try to maintain a balance. This is why weight gain is often the first symptom of Type 2 diabetes. But then we have to ask what causes insulin resistance to begin with, and many researchers believe that it is triggered by obesity. So it becomes a "chicken or egg" puzzle.

Many theories also surround the function of fat cells. Are some people genetically programmed to have more, or "fatter," fat cells than others? No answers here, yet.

What about the brain and obesity? Some propose that obesity is all in the head and has something to do with the hypothalamus (a part of the brain that controls messages to other parts of the body) somehow malfunctioning when it comes to sending the body the message "I'm full." It's believed that the hypothalamus may control satiation messages. To other researchers, the problem has to do with a defect in the body that doesn't recognize hunger cues or satiation cues, but the studies in this area are not conclusive.

A study reported in a 1997 issue of *Nature Medicine* showed that people with low levels of the hormone leptin may be prone to weight gain. In this study, people who gained an average of 50 pounds over three years started out with lower leptin levels than people who maintained their weight over the same period. Therefore, this study may form the basis for treating obesity with leptin. Experts speculate that 10 percent of all obesity may be due to leptin resistance. Leptin is made by fat cells and apparently sends messages to the brain about how much fat our bodies are carrying. Like other hormones, it's thought that leptin has a stimulating action that acts as a thermostat of sorts. In mice, adequate amounts of leptin somehow signaled the mouse to become more active and eat less, while too little leptin signaled the mouse to eat more while becoming less active.

Interestingly, Pima Indians in the United States, who are prone to obesity, were shown to have roughly one-third less leptin than the general population in blood analyses. Human studies of injecting leptin to treat obesity are in the works right now but to date have not been shown to be effective.

The U.S. government recently approved an antiobesity pill that blocks the absorption of almost one-third of the fat a person eats. One of the side effects of this new prescription drug, called orlistat (Xenical), causes rather embarrassing diarrhea each time you eat fatty foods. To avoid the drug's side effects, simply avoid fat! The pill can also decrease absorption of vitamin D and other important nutrients, however.

Orlistat is the first drug to fight obesity through the intestine instead of the brain. Taken with each meal, it binds to certain pancreatic enzymes to block the digestion of 30 percent of the fat you ingest. How it affects the pancreas in the long term is not known, however. Combined with a sensible diet, people on orlistat lost more weight than those not on it. This drug is not intended for people who need to lose only a few pounds; it is designed for medically obese people. (Orlistat was also found to lower cholesterol, blood pressure, and blood sugar levels.)

One of the most controversial antiobesity therapies was the use of fenfluramine and phentermine (Fen/Phen). Both drugs were approved for use individually more than twenty years ago, but since 1992, doctors prescribed them together for long-term management of obesity. (This is known as "off-label" prescribing.) In 1996, U.S. doctors wrote a total of 18 million monthly prescriptions for Fen/Phen. Many of the prescriptions were issued to people who were not medically obese. In July 1997, the U.S. Food and Drug Administration, researchers at the Mayo Clinic, and the Mayo Foundation made a joint announcement warning doctors that Fen/Phen can cause heart disease. On September 15, 1997, "Fen"(fenfluramine) was taken off the market. More bad news has surfaced about Fen/Phen wreaking havoc on serotonin levels, which only reinforces the message that in light of the safety concerns regarding current antiobesity drugs, diet and lifestyle modification are still considered the best pathways to wellness.

Overeating

When we hear "eating disorder," we usually think about anorexia or bulimia. Many people, however, binge without purging. This is also known as binge eating disorder or compulsive overeating. In this case, the bingeing is an announcement to the world that "I'm out of control." Someone who purges her bingeing behavior is hiding her lack of control. Someone who binges and never purges is advertising his lack of control. The purger is passively asking for help; the binger who doesn't purge is aggressively asking for help. It's the same disease with a different result. But there is one more layer when it comes to compulsive overeating, which is considered to be controversial and often rejected by the overeater: the desire to get fat is often behind the compulsion. Many people who overeat insist that fat is a consequence of eating food, not a goal. Many therapists who deal with overeating disagree and believe that if a woman admits that she has an emotional interest in actually being large, she may be much closer to stopping her compulsion to eat.

Furthermore, many women who eat compulsively do not recognize that they are doing so. The following is a typical profile of a compulsive eater:

- Eating when you're not hungry.

- Feeling out of control when you're around food, either trying to resist it or gorging on it.

- Spending a lot of time thinking/worrying about food and your weight.

- Always desperate to try another diet that promises results.

- Feelings of self-loathing and shame.

- Hating your own body.

- Obsessed with what you can or will eat, or have eaten.

- Eating in secret or with "eating friends."

- Appearing in public to be a professional dieter who's in control.

- Buying cakes or pies and having them wrapped as gifts to hide the fact that they're for you.

- Having a pristine kitchen with only the right foods.

- Feeling either out of control with food (compulsive eating), or imprisoned by it (dieting).

- Feeling temporary relief by not eating.

- Looking forward with pleasure and anticipation to the time when you can eat alone.

- Feeling unhappy because of your eating behavior.

Most people eat when they're hungry. But if you're a compulsive eater, hunger cues have nothing to do with when you eat.

You may eat for any of the following reasons:

- As a social event: this includes family meals, or meeting friends at restaurants. The point is that you plan food as the social entertainment. Most of us do this, but often we do it when we're not even hungry.
- To satisfy "mouth hunger"—the need to have something in the mouth, even though you are not hungry.
- Eating to prevent future hunger: "better eat now because later I may not get a chance."
- Eating as a reward for a bad day or bad experience; or to reward yourself for a good day or good experience.
- Eating because "it's the only pleasure I can count on!"
- Eating to quell nerves.
- Eating because you're bored.
- Eating now because you're going on a diet tomorrow. (Hence, the eating is done out of a real fear that you will be deprived later.)
- Eating because food is your friend.

Food addiction, like other addictions, can be treated successfully with a twelve-step program. For those of you who aren't familiar with this type of program, I've provided the text of "The Twelve Steps." The twelve-step program was started in the 1930s by an alcoholic who was able to overcome his addiction by essentially saying, "God, help me!" He found other alcoholics who were in a similar position and through an organized, nonjudgmental support system, they overcame their addiction by realizing that God (a higher power, spirit, force, physical properties of the universe, or intelligence) helps those who help themselves. In other words, you have to want the help. This is the premise of Alcoholics Anonymous—the most successful recovery program for addicts that exists.

People with other addictions have adopted the same program, using Alcoholics Anonymous and the "The Twelve Steps and Twelve Traditions," the founding literature for Alcoholics Anonymous. Overeaters Anonymous substitutes the phrase "compulsive overeater" for "alcoholic" and "food" for "alcohol." The theme of all twelve-step programs is best ex-pressed through the Serenity Prayer: "God grant me the serenity to accept the things I cannot change, the courage to change the things I can, and the wisdom to know the difference." In other words, you can't take back the food you ate yesterday or last year; but you can control the food you eat today instead of feeling guilty about yesterday.

Every twelve-step program also has "The Twelve Traditions," which, essentially, is a code of conduct. To join an OA program, you need only to take the first step. Abstinence and the next two steps are what most people are able to do in six to twelve months before moving on. In an OA program, abstinence means three meals daily, weighed and measured, with nothing in between except sugar-free or no-calorie beverages and sugar-free gum. Your food is written down and called in. The program also advises you to get your doctor's approval before starting. Abstinence is continued through a continuous process of "one day at a time" and sponsors—people who call you to check in and who you can call when the cravings hit. Sponsors are recovering overeaters who have been there and who can talk you through your cravings.

OA membership is predominantly female; if you are interested in joining OA and are male, you may feel more comfortable in an all-male group. Many women overeaters overeat because they have been harmed by men, and their anger is often directed at the one male in the room; this may not be a comfortable position for a male overeater. For this reason, OA is now divided into all-female and all-male groups.

The Twelve Steps of Overeaters Anonymous

Step One: I admit I am powerless over food and that my life has become unmanageable.

Step Two: I've come to believe that a Power greater than myself can restore me to sanity.

Step Three: I've made a decision to turn my will and my life over to the care of a Higher Power, as I understand it.

Step Four: I've made a searching and fearless moral inventory of myself.

Step Five: I've admitted to a Higher Power, to myself, and to another human being the exact nature of my wrongs.

Step Six: I'm entirely ready to have a Higher Power remove all these defects of character.

Step Seven: I've humbly asked a Higher Power to remove my shortcomings.

Step Eight: I've made a list of all persons I have harmed and have become willing to make amends to them all.

Step Nine: I've made direct amends to such people wherever possible, except when to do so would injure them or others.

Step Ten: I've continued to take personal inventory and when I was wrong, promptly admitted it.

Step Eleven: I've sought through prayer and meditation to improve my conscious contact with a Higher Power, as I understand it, praying only for knowledge of Its will for me and the power to carry that out.

Step Twelve: Having had a spiritual awakening as the result of these steps, I've tried to carry this message to compulsive overeaters and to practice these principles in all my affairs.

44. Cut the Caffeine

Caffeine is hard on the gut, and by cutting it down or out, many people find their upper G.I. symptoms improve. Here's a checklist of how much caffeine some foods contain, with the milligrams of caffeine in parentheses:

Coffee (5-ounce cup)

Brewed, drip method	(60–180)
Brewed, percolator	(40–170)
Instant	(30–120)
Decaffeinated, brewed	(2–5)
Decaffeinated, instant	(1–5)

Tea (5-ounce cup)

Brewed, major brands	(20–90)
Brewed, imported brands	(25–110)
Instant	(25–50)
12-ounce glass, iced	(67–76)

Other

6-ounce glass of caffeine-containing soft drink	(15–30)
5-ounce cup of cocoa beverage	(2–20)
8-ounce glass of chocolate milk	(2–7)
1-ounce serving of milk chocolate	(1–15)
1-ounce serving of dark chocolate, semisweet	(5–35)
Single square of Baker's chocolate	(26)
Serving of chocolate-flavored syrup	(4)

45. Add the Fiber

Fiber is vital for avoiding constipation. Fiber is the part of a plant your body can't digest. It comes in the form of water-soluble fiber (which dissolves in water) and water-insoluble fiber (which does not dissolve in water but instead, absorbs water); this is what's meant by soluble and insoluble fiber. Soluble and insoluble fiber do differ, but they are equally beneficial.

Soluble fiber somehow lowers the bad cholesterol, or low-density lipids (LDL), in your body. Experts aren't entirely sure how soluble fiber works its magic, but one popular theory is that it gets mixed into the bile the liver secretes and forms a type of gel that traps the building blocks of cholesterol, thus lowering your LDL levels. It's akin to a spider trapping smaller insects in its web.

Insoluble fiber doesn't affect your cholesterol levels at all, but it regulates your bowel movements. How does it do this? As insoluble fiber moves through your digestive tract, it absorbs water like a sponge and helps to form waste into a solid form fast, making the stools large, soft, and easy to pass. Without insoluble fiber, solid waste just gets pushed down to the colon or lower intestine as always, where it is stored and dried out until you're ready to have a bowel movement. High-starch foods are associated with dry stools. This is exacerbated when you "ignore the urge," as the colon dehydrates the waste even more until it becomes hard and difficult to pass, a condition known as constipation. Insoluble fiber helps regulate bowel movements by speeding things along. Insoluble fiber increases the transit time by increasing colon motility and limiting the time dietary toxins hang around the intestinal wall. This is why it can dramatically decrease your risk of colon cancer.

Sources of Insoluble Fiber

Good sources of insoluble fiber are wheat bran and whole grains, skins from various fruits and vegetables, seeds, leafy greens, and cruciferous vegetables (cauliflower, broccoli, and brussels sprouts). The problem is understanding what is truly whole grain. For example, there is an assumption that because bread is dark or brown, it's more nutritious; this isn't so. In fact, many brown breads are simply enriched white breads dyed with molasses. ("Enriched" means that nutrients lost during processing have been replaced.) High-fiber pita breads and bagels are available, but you have to search for them. A good rule is to simply look for the phrase "whole wheat," which means that the wheat is, indeed, whole.

Most of us turn to grains and cereals to boost our fiber intake, which experts recommend should be about 25 to 35 grams per day. Use Table 45.1 to help gauge whether you're getting enough. The following list indicates the amount of insoluble fiber in various foods. If you're a little under par, an easy way to boost your fiber intake is to simply add pure wheat bran to your foods. It is available in health food stores or supermarkets in a sort of sawdust-like form. Three table-

Table 45.1

Cereals (based on ½ cup unless otherwise specified)	Grams of fiber
Fiber First	15.0
Fiber One	12.8
All Bran	10.0
Oatmeal (1 cup)	5.0
Raisin Bran (¾ cup)	4.6
Bran Flakes (1 cup)	4.4
Shreddies (⅔ cup)	2.7
Cheerios (1 cup)	2.2
Corn Flakes (1¼ cup)	0.8
Special K (1 cup)	0.4
Rice Krispies (1¼ cup)	0.3

Breads (based on 1 slice)	Grams of fiber
Rye	2.0
Pumpernickel	2.0
Twelve grain	1.7
100% whole wheat	1.3
Raisin	1.0
Cracked wheat	1.0
White	0

spoons of wheat bran provide 4.4 grams of fiber. Sprinkle 1 to 2 tablespoons onto cereals, rice, pasta, or meat dishes. You can also sprinkle it into orange juice or low-fat yogurt. It has virtually no calories. It's important to drink a glass of water with your wheat bran, as well a glass of water after you've finished your wheat bran–enriched meal.

Keep in mind that some of the new high-fiber breads on the market today have up to 7 grams of fiber per slice. Table 45.1 is based on what is normally found in typical grocery stores.

Drink Water with Fiber

Think of fiber as a sponge. Obviously, a dry sponge won't work. You must soak it with water for it to be useful—same thing here. Fiber without water is as useful as a dry sponge. You must soak your fiber! So here is the fiber/water recipe:

- Drink two glasses of water with your fiber. This means having a glass of water with whatever you're eating. Even if what you're eating does not contain much fiber, drinking water with your meal is a good habit to get into!

- Drink two glasses of water after you eat.

46. Get Moving

Gravity helps your food go down. You have to get off the couch and move if you want your G.I. symptoms to improve without drug therapy. Reports from the United States show that one out of three American adults is overweight, a sign of growing inactivity. The fitness industry has a done an excellent job of intimidating inactive people. Some people are so put off by the health club scene, they become even more sedentary. This is similar to diet failure, where you become so demoralized that you "cheat" and binge even more.

What's the definition of sedentary? Not moving! If you have a desk job or spend most of your time at a computer, in your car, or watching television (even if it is PBS or CNN), you are a sedentary person. If you do roughly twenty minutes of exercise less than once a week, you're relatively sedentary. You need to incorporate some sort of movement into your daily schedule to be considered active. That movement can be anything: aerobic exercise, brisk walks around the block, or walking your dog. If you've been sedentary most of your life, there's nothing wrong with starting off with simple, even leisurely activities such as gardening, feeding the birds in a park, or a few simple stretches. Any step you take toward being more active is a crucial and important one. A 1998 *New England Journal of Medicine* article reported that low-intensity exercises such as walking were associated with lower rates of cancers, such as colon cancer and prostate cancer.

Experts also recommend that you find a friend, neighbor, or relative to "get physical" with you. When your exercise plans include someone else, you'll be less apt to cancel them or make excuses for not getting out there.

Choose an activity that's right for you (see Table 46.1). Whether it's walking, chopping wood, jumping rope, or folk dancing—pick something you enjoy. You don't have to do the same thing each time, either. Vary your routine to avoid monotony. Just make sure that whatever activity you choose is continuous. Walking for two minutes, then stopping for three isn't continuous. It's also important to choose an activity that doesn't aggravate a preexisting health problem. Try not to let two days pass without doing something.

Table 46.1 Suggested Activities

More intense	Less intense
Skiing	Golf
Running	Bowling
Jogging	Badminton
Stair stepping or stair climbing	Croquet
Trampolining	Sailing
Jumping rope	Strolling
Fitness walking	Stetching
Race walking	
Aerobic classes	
Roller skating	
Ice skating	
Biking	
Weight-lifting exercises	
Tennis	
Swimming	

Also, pick a length of time to exercise. If you're elderly or ill, even a few minutes is a good start. If you're sedentary but otherwise healthy, aim for twenty to thirty minutes.

The Meaning of Exercise

The *Oxford English Dictionary* defines exercise as "the exertion of muscles, limbs, etc., especially for health's sake; bodily, mental, or spiritual training." In the Western world, we have placed an emphasis on "bodily training" when we talk about exercise, completely ignoring mental and spiritual training. Only recently have Western studies begun to focus on the mental benefits of exercise. (It's been shown, for example, that exercise creates endorphins, hormones that make us feel good.) But we in the West do not encourage meditation or other calming forms of mental and spiritual exercise, which have also been shown to improve well-being and health, particularly by reducing stress—a major risk factor for heart disease.

In the East, for thousands of years, exercise has focused on achieving mental and spiritual health through the body, using breathing and postures, for example. Nor should we ignore cultural traditions known to improve mental health and well-being, such as traditional dances, active prayers that incorporate physical activity, circles that involve community and communication, and sweat lodges, believed to help rid the body of toxins through sweating. These are all forms of wellness activities that you should investigate.

If you look up the word *aerobic* in the dictionary, what you'll find is the chemistry definition: "living in free oxygen." This is certainly correct; we are all aerobes—beings that require oxygen to live. Some bacteria, for example, are anaerobic; they can exist in an environment without oxygen. All that jumping around and fast movement is done to create faster breathing, so we can take more oxygen into our bodies.

Why are we doing this? Because the blood contains oxygen! The faster your blood flows, the more oxygen can flow to your organs. But when your health care practitioner tells you to exercise or to take up aerobic exercise he is not referring solely to increasing oxygen but to exercising the heart muscle. The faster it beats, the better a workout it gets. If you already have heart disease, or are on medications that affect your heart, check with your doctor to make sure you do not overwork your heart.

When more oxygen is in our bodies, we burn fat (see below), our breathing improves, our blood pressure improves, and our hearts work better. Oxygen also lowers triglycerides and cholesterol, increasing our high-density lipoproteins (HDL) or the good cholesterol, while decreasing our low-density lipoproteins (LDL) or the bad cholesterol. This means that your arteries will unclog and you may significantly decrease your risk of heart disease and stroke. More oxygen makes our brains work better, so we feel better. Studies show that depression is decreased when we increase oxygen flow into our bodies. Ancient techniques such as yoga, which specifically improve mental and spiritual well-being, achieve this by combining deep breathing and stretching, which improves oxygen and blood flow to specific parts of the body.

Exercise has been shown to dramatically decrease the incidence of many other diseases, including cancer. Some research suggests that cancer cells tend to thrive in an oxygen-depleted environment. The more oxygen in the bloodstream, the less hospitable you make your body to cancer. In addition, since many cancers are related to fat-soluble toxins, the less fat on your body, the less fat-soluble toxins your body can accumulate.

A way to measure exercise intensity without finding your pulse, is Borg's Rate of Perceived (RPE), now the recommended method for judging exertion. This Borg scale, as it's dubbed, goes from 6 to 20. Extremely light activity may rate a 7, for example, while a very intense activity may rate a 19. Exercise practitioners recommend that you do a "talk test" to rate your exertion, too. If you can't talk without gasping for air, you may be working too hard. You should be able to carry on a normal conversation throughout your activity. What's crucial to remember about RPE is that it is extremely subjective; what one person judges a 7, another may judge a 10.

47. Stretches Good for the Gut

To help your food go down, here are some interesting, yet challenging yoga stretches to try:

- Locust. Lie on your belly with your arms folded beneath you, palms pressed into your body. Extend both legs until they lift up and off the floor. Keep the toes pointed. Release.

- Cobra (Upward Facing Dog). Lie on your belly with your palms down and adjacent to your shoulders. Slowly raise your upper body, lifting all but the lower abdomen toward the ceiling. Breathe deeply. Release.

- Fish. Lie on your back. Place your hands under your sitting bones, palms pressed into the floor, feet flexed. Gently roll one, then the other shoulder inward, shortening the distance between your shoulder blades (your chest will naturally arch upwards). Breathe, lengthening your abdominals and rib cage. Release.

There are also stretches you can do to help strengthen your abdominal muscles, which can help to combat constipation:

- The Squat. As shown in Figure 47.1, by doing this regularly, you can become more regular, too! Stand with your feet parallel to your hips and slowly squat down, making sure your weight is forward (rather than reeling backward); avoid rolling your knees inward. You may need to practice a few times before you can do this comfortably. It's recommended that you squat twice a day to aid constipation.

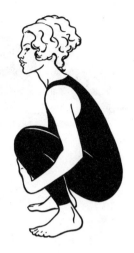

FIGURE 47.1

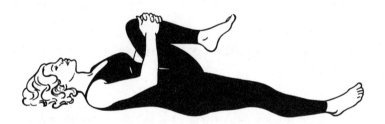

FIGURE 47.2

- Knee-to-chest—one leg. As shown in Figure 47.2, this strengthens your abdominal muscles and, when combined with the squat (see Figure 47.1), can beautifully relieve chronic constipation. Lie on your back on the floor. Bend one knee and bring it in to the chest. Then just hug the leg, and slowly bring it toward your

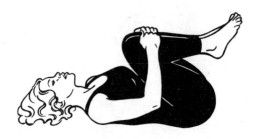

FIGURE 47.3

abdomen. Hold for a count of 10. Relax and repeat
with alternate leg.

- Knee-to-chest—both legs. As shown in Figure 47.3,
  this is the same as the one-leg version, only you bring
  both legs to the chest and hug them with both arms,
  bringing them gently toward your abdomen. Hold
  them there for the count of 10. Then relax and repeat.

48. Incorporate Active Living

There are many ways you can adopt an active lifestyle.
Here are some suggestions:

- If you drive everywhere, pick the parking space fur-
  thest from your destination so you can work some
  daily walking into your life.

- If you take public transit everywhere, get off one or
  two stops early so you can walk the rest of the way
  to your destination.

- Choose stairs often over escalators or elevators.

- Park at one side of the mall and then walk to the
  other.

- Take a stroll around your neighborhood after dinner.
- Volunteer to walk the dog.
- On weekends, go to the zoo or get out to flea markets, garage sales, and so on.
- Other suggested activities are listed in Table 46.1 on page 101.

Getting creative is also a way of motivating yourself. For example, try some of these variations on jogging:

- After warming up with a fifteen-minute walk, walk quickly with maximum exertion for two minutes, then slow down for one minute. Keep your heart rate up on the downhill portion of a walk or a hike by adding lunges or squats.
- Vary the way you walk for coordination and balance. Try lifting the knees as high as you can, as if marching. Alternate with a shuffle, letting the tips of your fingers touch the ground as you walk. Do a sideways crab walk. To strengthen the rarely used muscles of the ankles and feet, walk first on the outsides, then on the insides of your feet. Or practice walking backwards.
- Use a curb for a step workout. Or climb stairs two at a time.

Water Workouts

- Start by walking in water that's relatively shallow (waist or chest deep). Your breathing and heartbeat will determine how hard you are working. Since you'll be moving fairly slowly, pay attention to your body.

- For all-over leg toning, take fifty steps forward, fifty steps sideways in crablike fashion, fifty steps backward, then fifty steps to the other side.

- To tone your arms, submerge yourself from the neck down, bringing the arms in and out as if clapping. The water provides natural resistance.

- Deep-water workouts are the most difficult because every move you make is met with resistance. Wear a flotation vest and run without touching the bottom for optimum exertion and little or no impact.

- You may also want to try buoyant ankle cuffs and Styrofoam dumbbells or kickboards for full-body conditioning in the water.

Deep Breathing

- Deep relaxation and yoga breathing, such as alternate nostril breath, calms the sympathetic nervous system, thus relaxing the small arteries and lowering blood pressure.

49. Understand the Role of Stress

Experts cite stress as a leading cause of many upper and lower G.I. problems. Your G.I. tract is controlled by your nervous system, which is why it reacts when you're under stress. In the same way that you can sweat, blush, or cry under emotional stress, your G.I. tract may also react to stress by "weeping"—producing excessive water and mucus and overreacting to normal stimuli such as eating. What often happens, however, is that there is a delayed "gut reaction" to stress, and you may not experience your G.I. symptoms until your stress has passed. Apparently, under stress your brain becomes more active as a defense. (For example, when we're running away from a predator, we have to think quickly and act quickly, so our heart rates increase, we sweat more, and so on.) During this defensive mode the entire nervous system can become exaggerated (that's what causes "butterflies in the stomach"). The nerves controlling the G.I. tract therefore become highly sensitive, which can cause an array of G.I. symptoms.

In response to stress, your adrenal glands pump out stress hormones that speed up your body: Your heart rate increases, and your blood sugar levels increase so that glucose can be diverted to your muscles in case you have to run. This is known as the "fight or flight" response. The problem with stress hormones in the twenty-first century is that the fight or flight response isn't usually necessary, since most of our stress is emotional. Occasionally, we may want to flee from a bank robber or a mugger, but most of us just want to flee from our jobs or our kids! In other words, our stress hormones actually put a physical strain on our bodies and can lower our resistance to disease, which can impact our bodies from head to toe. We can suffer from stress-related:

- Headaches.
- Gastrointestinal problems.
- Bladder problems.
- Heart problems.
- Back pain.
- High blood pressure.
- High cholesterol.

Good Stress

Good things come from good stress, even though it feels stressful or bad in the short term. Stress challenges us to stretch ourselves beyond our capabilities, which is what makes us meet deadlines, push the outside of the envelope, and invent creative solutions to our problems. Examples of good stress include challenging projects; positive life-changing events (moving, changing jobs, or ending unhealthy relationships); confronting fears, illness, or people who make us feel bad (this is one of those bad-in-the-short-term but good-in-the-long-term situations). Essentially, whenever a stressful event triggers emotional, intellectual, or spiritual growth, it is a good stress. It is often not the event as much as your response to it that determines whether it is a good or bad stress. The death of a loved one can sometimes lead to personal growth because we may see something about ourselves we did not see before—new resilience, for example. So even a death can be a good stress, though we grieve and are sad in the short term.

Bad Stress

Bad stress results from boredom and stagnation. When no growth occurs from a stressful event, it is bad stress. When negative events don't seem to yield anything positive in the long term except more of the same, the stress can lead to chronic and debilitating health problems. This is not to say that we can't get sick from good stress, either, but when nothing positive results, stress has a much more negative effect on our health. Some examples of bad stress include stagnant jobs or relationships, disability caused by terrible accidents or diseases, or long-term unemployment. These kinds of situations can lead to depression, low self-esteem, and a host of physical illnesses.

Managing Stress

What we perceive as stressful has great bearing on how well we manage it. Women that are already overloaded will feel additional stress as well. In general, we feel stress when we experience:

- Negative events.

- Uncontrollable or unpredictable events.

- Ambiguous events (versus clear-cut situations).

How stressed you become has much to do with your personality as well. For example, if you have a negative outlook on life, you'll probably feel more stress than someone with a positive outlook. Some like to find meaning in uncontrollable events, which gives them a sense of control. Others like the challenge of difficult situations.

Our coping strategies also vary. Some like to avoid stress and minimize the problem. This has short-term benefits but, in the long term, the stress does not disappear. People who confront stressors in the short term will feel more anxious at first but will probably feel relief in the long term when it is dealt with. People who use humor, spiritual support, and social support to deal with stress suffer fewer stress-related health problems.

Stress reduction entirely depends on the source of your stress. The only way to control stress that is beyond your control is to shift your response to it. For many, this takes time and may require some work with a qualified counselor.

If you are the source of your own stress because you're too hard on yourself, or are a perfectionist, you need to work on lowering your self-expectations and forgiving yourself for not being perfect. Again, working with a therapist or counselor may help.

If the following statements sound like you, you're probably not managing stress very well:

- I tend to imagine all the terrible things that could
  possibly happen to me rather than just concerning
  myself with the stressful situation at hand.

- I stop what I'm doing and devote all my energy
  toward fixing a problem immediately. (I might as
  well do this because, if I don't, I will just drive
  myself crazy with worry.)

- I relive my latest crisis in my mind over and over
  again—even after it's been solved.

- I actually picture the stressful situation in my mind's
  eye, as well as picturing the worst possible outcome.

- I get the feeling that I'm losing control over
  everything.

- I have a sinking feeling in my stomach; I feel my
  mouth getting dry, my heart pounding, or my neck
  and shoulder muscles tightening.

- I have trouble falling asleep at night, and I wake up
  in the middle of the night.

- I tend to make mountains out of molehills. (I sort of
  know I'm doing this, but I can't stop myself.)

- I have difficulty speaking or notice my hands and/or
  fingers trembling.

- I notice my thoughts racing.

Here are a number of suggestions for reducing some
sources of daily stress:

- Isolate the exact source of stress and see if there's a
  solution. (Taking the time to think about what, in
  fact, the real problem is can work wonders.)

- See the humor in difficult situations and try to look at lessons learned instead of beating yourself up.

- When times get tough, surround yourself with supportive people: close friends, family members, and so on.

- Don't take things personally. When people don't respond to you the way you'd like, consider other factors. For instance, maybe the other person has problems unrelated to you that are affecting his behavior.

- Focus on something pleasant in the future, such as a vacation, and allow yourself time to daydream, plan, and so on.

- Just say no. If you can't take on that small favor or extra task, just politely say, "I'd love to, but it's impossible."

- Take time out for yourself. Spend some time alone and block everyone out once a week or so. This is a great time to just go for a long walk and get in a little exercise.

- Make lists. Some people find list making really helps; others find it is just another chore in and of itself. But if you haven't been a list maker, try it. It might help you get a little more focused and organized on the tasks at hand.

- Look at some alternative healing systems, such as massage or Chinese exercises, qi gong (pronounced chi kong) or tai chi.

- Eat properly.

Finding a Good Stress Counselor or Therapist

In your hunt for a counselor to work with you on reducing stress, any of the following professionals can help:

- Psychiatrist. This is a medical doctor who specializes in the medical treatment of mental illness and is able to prescribe drugs. Many psychiatrists also do psychotherapy, but this isn't always the case. The appropriate credentials should read: Jane Doe, M.D. (medical doctor), F.A.C.P. (Fellow, American College of Physicians); in Canada, F.R.C.P. (Fellow, Royal College of Physicians). That means this doctor has gone through four years of medical school and has completed a residency program in psychiatry, which, depending on the state, lasted approximately four years, and is registered in the American College of Physicians and Surgeons. (Or, if trained in Canada or the United Kingdom, the Royal College of Physicians and Surgeons.)

- Psychologist or psychological associate. This is someone who can be licensed to practice therapy with either a master's degree or doctoral degree. Clinical psychologists have a master of science degree (MSc.) or master of arts (MA), and usually work in a hospital or clinic setting but often are in private practice. Clinical psychologists can also hold a Ph.D. (Doctor of Philosophy) in psychology, an Ed.D. (Doctor of Education) or, if they're American, a Psy.D. (Doctor of Psychology), a common degree in the United States. Psychologists often perform testing and assessments and plan treatments. They can also do psychotherapy, may have hospital admitting privileges, and should be registered with their state licensing board. Licensure is required in all fifty states. Licensure requirements are generally uniform across states, authorizing the psychologist to independently diagnose and treat mental and nervous disorders on completion of both a doctoral degree in psychology (Ph.D., Psy.D., or Ed.D.) and a minimum of two years of supervised experience in direct clinical service. In some states, psychologists can also prescribe drugs.

- Social worker. This professional holds a BSW (bachelor of social work) and/or a MSW (master of social work), having completed a bachelor's degree in another discipline (which is not at all uncommon). Some social workers have Ph.D.s as well. A professional social worker has a degree in social work and meets state legal requirements. The designation CSW stands for certified social worker. It is a legal title granted by the state. A designation of ACSW refers to the National Association of Social Worker's (NASW) own, nongovernmental national credential and stands for the Academy of Certified Social Workers. Unlike the CSW, which in addition to the exam requires graduation (in most states) from a master's level program, the ACSW requires two years of supervised experience following graduation from such a program. Some social workers have a "P" and "R"; these letters stand for CSWs who have become qualified under state law to receive insurance reimbursement for outpatient services to clients with group health insurance. Each initial refers to different types of insurance policies. The "P" requires three years of supervised experience, while the "R" requires six years.

- Psychiatric nurse. This is most likely a registered nurse (R.N.) with a bachelor of science degree in nursing (BSc.) (not absolutely required) who probably has, but doesn't necessarily require, a master's degree in nursing, too. The master's degree could be either an MA (master of arts) or an MSc. (master of science). This nurse has done most of her training in a psychiatric setting and may be trained to do psychotherapy.

- Counselor. This professional has usually completed certification courses in counseling and therefore has obtained a license to practice psychotherapy; he may have, but does not require, a university degree. Frequently, though, counselors will have a master's degree in a related field, such as social work. Or, they may have a master's degree in a field having nothing to do with mental health. The term *professional counselor* is used to represent those persons who have earned a minimum of a master's degree and possess professional knowledge and demonstrable skills in the application of mental health, psychological, and human development principles to facilitate human development and adjustment throughout a person's life span. As of January 1999, the District of Columbia and forty-four states have enacted some type of counselor credentialing law that regulates the use of titles related to the counseling profession. The letters "CPC" stand for certified professional counselor and refer to the title granted by the state legislative process. The letters "LPC" stand for licensed professional counselor and refer to the most often granted state statutory counselor credential. No matter what letters you see, however, it's always a good idea to ask your counselor what training she has had in the field of mental health.

- Marriage and family counselor. This is somewhat different than the broader term *counselor*. This professional has completed rigorous training through certification courses in family therapy and relationship dynamics and has obtained a license to practice psychotherapy. This professional should have the designations MFT or AAFMT. MFTs have graduate training (a master's or doctoral degree) in marriage and family therapy and at least two years of clinical experience. There are forty-one states currently licensing, certifying, or regulating MFTs.

It's important to discuss fees with your therapist up front, so you know what services are covered by your health plan. In general, mental health services in hospitals are covered by health plans, as are services provided by psychiatrists. Social workers or counselors in private practice are all fee for service, however. Call the National Association of Social Workers (NASW) at 1-800-638-8799 to determine what a social worker or counselor in private practice should be charging and to obtain a copy of the NASW Code of Ethics. If you want to see someone in private practice but can't afford to pay, some community-provided counseling services are based on your ability to pay. Experts consulted for this book agreed that it is considered bad practice for a counselor to agree to see someone who cannot (or will not) pay for his services. This person is offering a service, not a charity, and the professional relationship should be respected. As of this writing, psychiatrists typically charge roughly $100 to $175 per hour/session; clinical psychologists charge roughly $85 to $120 per hour/session, and social workers charge $65 to $110 per hour/session.

If you have health coverage through a managed care plan, you may be in for a rude awakening when it comes to coverage of psychiatric services. Most plans cover only thirty days of inpatient psychiatric care per year and twenty outpatient visits to a psychotherapist. This is fine if you require only short-term therapy, but for most people suffering from depression or mood disorders, this coverage is inadequate. Some plans offer "conversion of benefits," meaning that you can convert your thirty days of inpatient coverage to thirty extra days of outpatient visits, giving you sixty outpatient visits covered.

An extremely important consideration for anyone having psychiatric services covered by a health insurance plan is confidentiality. Managed care facilities require frequent record reviews by psychiatric service providers, which means that confidentiality between you and your mental health care provider may be compromised. Discuss this aspect of treatment when you discuss fees and costs; it's important.

Going for a Test Drive

Okay. You found someone you think is qualified to be your therapist. That doesn't mean you found the right therapist for you. Ask yourself the following questions when you first sit down with this therapist. If you find you answer no to many of the questions below, you should consider whether you're really with the right therapist. There is no magic number of no's here; but these questions will help you gauge how you truly feel about this professional.

- Is this someone with whom you feel comfortable?
- Is this someone you can trust?
- Is this someone with whom you feel calm?

- Is this someone with whom you feel safe?
- Does this person respect you (or treat you with respect)?
- Does this person seem flexible?
- Does this person seem reliable?
- Does this person seem supportive?
- Does this person have a supervisor or mentor with whom she consults on difficult or challenging cases?

50. Use Spices Good for Digestion

- Coriander. Eases gases and works to tone the digestive system. Use powdered or whole seed, or garnish with fresh leaves (cilantro).
- Cardamom. Reduces the mucus-forming effects of dairy products. Use powdered or whole seeds.
- Turmeric. Generally improves metabolism and helps you to digest proteins. Use the ground root. (Gives dishes a yellowish color and can stain clothes and china.)
- Black pepper. Stimulates appetite and helps you digest dairy products. Use freshly ground.
- Cumin. Helps reduce gases and generally tones the digestive system. Use seeds whole or powdered.
- Fennel. Helps prevent gas. Chew the seeds after eating, or add them to vegetables that tend to produce gas when cooked. Use whole or powdered.
- Ginger. Aids digestion and respiration. Also helps to relieve gas and constipation, or indigestion. Use root

fresh or dried. (Note: ginger can aggravate bleeding ulcers.)

- Cinnamon. This naturally cleanses your digestive system. Use powdered, in sticks, or pieces.

- Nutmeg. This helps your body absorb nutrients from food, but should be used sparingly.

- Clove. This also helps your body absorb nutrients. Use whole or ground.

- Cayenne. This helps to simulate your digestive juices and is known for having a cleansing action within the large intestine. Helps to relieve that feeling of fullness after eating a heavy meal.

Epilogue

This book is designed to help you stomach life on Earth a little better. You've learned about some of the first signs of serious G.I. problems, which often start with heartburn/reflux (Items 1 through 10); you may have gotten to the bottom of nagging symptoms that turn out to be ulcers (Items 11 through 20) or gastroesophageal reflux disease (Items 21 through 30). You also may have found that the source of your discomforts are linked to certain medications or that you're overdoing it on over-the-counter tummy medications (Items 31 through 40). But many of you will find simple relief from your chronic upper G.I. symptoms by making some changes to your lifestyle, such as quitting smoking, losing a bit of weight, and becoming more active (Items 41 through 50). If someone you know is suffering from chronic G.I. symptoms, you hold in your hands fifty ways to spell R-E-L-I-E-F.

Glossary

Note: This list is not exhaustive. These are not literal dictionary definitions but, rather, definitions created solely for the context of this book. Any resemblance to definitions found in other glossaries or dictionaries is purely coincidental.

Antacids: Medicines that relieve heartburn as well as peptic ulcer disease symptoms by neutralizing the stomach acid that rises up into the esophagus.

Barium enema: A chalky solution inserted into the colon that shows up on X-ray film.

Barret's esophagus: An ulcer located in the lining of the esophagus caused by the presence of acid in an area where it doesn't belong.

Bernstein test: A test for acidity to determine whether or not symptoms are a result of contact between the esophageal lining and acid.

Chronic symptoms: Symptoms that are experienced on a regular basis.

Digestion: The process by which food is converted into the nutrients we need to live and the excess waste we don't need.

Digestive hormones: Hormones that control the function of the digestive system and are secreted by the cells that line the stomach and small intestine.

Digestive system: A series of tubing, about twenty-two feet long, that twists and turns from the mouth to the anus.

Dysmotility: Impaired movement. In this case, impaired movement of some of the muscles in the G.I. tract.

Dysphagia: Difficulty swallowing caused by a blockage of food or liquid in the throat.

Early satiety: Feeling full after only a few bites.

Endoscopy: A test for esophagitis caused by heartburn. A thin, lighted tube is passed down the throat and the esophagus.

Esophageal manometry: A test that measures the pressure or tension of liquids in the esophagus.

Esophagitis: Inflammation of the esophageal lining.

Gastric emptying: The "juices and motion" segment of digestion, in which digestive juices, combined with the natural contractions and waves of all the tubing along the G.I. tract, move food from point A to point B.

Gastrin: A digestive hormone that signals the stomach to produce acid, necessary for the breakdown of food. Gastrin also controls the normal growth of cells and tissue in the stomach lining, small intestine, and colon.

Gastritis: Inflammation of the stomach lining.

Gastroenterologist: A gastrointestinal, or G.I., specialist.

Gastroesophageal reflux disease (GERD): Also called hypomotility, this condition occurs as a result of dysmotility and is characterized by a lack of sufficient contraction of the sphincter at the bottom of the esophagus, causing food mixed with stomach acid to come back up.

H2 receptor antagonist: A medication that inhibits the stomach from secreting acid. Used mainly as a pain reliever rather than a drug that treats an underlying problem.

Helicobacter pylori (H. pylori): A bacteria now believed to be the cause of ulcers. *H. pylori* lives in the stomach's mucus lining, causing it to slowly wear out.

Lactose intolerance: An allergy to milk caused by an absence of the enzyme lactase, which breaks down the sugar lactose into glucose.

Lower esophageal sphincter (LES): The crucial tunnel bridging the esophagus and the stomach, which acts as a ring-like valve that opens and closes, allowing food to pass.

Motility disorder: Occurs when the muscles in the esophagus and stomach region aren't coordinating well enough to move food from point A to point B.

Motility: The continuous movement characteristic of the process of gastric emptying, which is controlled by nerves, hormones, and muscles.

Non-ulcer dyspepsia (NUD): Discomfort in the upper G.I. tract not related to ulcer. NUD's symptoms, however, are completely indistinguishable from those of ulcers and heartburn.

Peptic ulcer disease (PUD): A disease that causes a very specific, localized area of pain in the upper G.I. tract because of a sore in the stomach lining.

Prokinetic drug: A drug that regulates the muscles in the G.I. tract by telling the brain to send the right messages to the muscles that control the G.I. tract. Prokinetic drugs help food get from the esophagus into the stomach, and then from the stomach into the small intestine. They do so by improving LES pressure and peristalsis, which gets rid of the acid in the esophagus and improves gastric emptying.

Proton pump inhibitor: A strong, acid-controlling drug such as lansoprazole.

Reflux: A fancy word for heartburn or acid indigestion, in which semidigested food comes back up the esophageal sphincter, causing a bitter taste in the mouth and a burning sensation in the esophagus. Reflux is usually a symptom of either GERD or ulcer.

Regurgitation: The coming back up of semidigested food.

Scintigraphy: A gastric emptying test that involves eating radioactive eggs that have been scrambled with technetium. A gamma counter then determines how quickly the scrambled eggs empty out of the stomach.

Secretin: A digestive hormone that kick-starts all the pancreatic juices, which contain bicarbonate. Secretin also signals the stomach to produce pepsin (which breaks down protein) and the liver to produce bile (which breaks down fat).

Small intestine: The midgut or small bowel. The small intestine can also be categorized as the duodenum, jejunum, and ileum.

Sodium bicarbonate: An alkaline substance in the duodenum that neutralizes stomach acid.

Stomach: An accordionlike bag of muscle and other tissue near the center of the abdomen just below the rib cage. The bag extends to accommodate food and shrinks when it is empty. The stomach itself is a "holding tank" for food until it can be distributed into more distant parts of the gastrointestinal tract.

Ulcer crater: The inflamed area surrounding an ulcer.

Ulcer: Occurs when a small surface of an organ or tissue has sloughed off, resulting in a sore.

Upper G.I. series: A diagnostic test that involves taking a series of images followed by a barium tracer to determine what's going on in the upper G.I. tract.

Upper G.I. tract: Everything above the large intestine.

Where to Go for More Information

United States

Celiac Sprue Association of the United States of America
(CSAUSA)
P.O. Box 700
Omaha, NE 68131-0700
(402) 558-0600
Fax: (402) 558-1347
Email: celiacusa@aol.com

National Digestive Diseases Information Clearinghouse
2 Information Way
Bethesda, MD 20892-3570

American Anorexia & Bulimia Society (AABA)
293 Central Park West, #1R
New York, NY 10024
(212) 501-8351

National Association for Anorexia Nervosa and
Associated Disorders
P.O. Box 7
Highland Park, Il 60035
(847) 831-3438

Anorexia Nervosa and Related Eating Disorders, Inc.
    P.O. Box 5102
    Eugene, OR 97405
    (503) 344-1144

Overeaters Anonymous (OA)
    Head Office:
    World Services Offices
    P.O. Box 44020
    Rio Rancho, NM 87124

Hotlines

American Dietetic Association and National Center for
    Nutrition and Dietetics (NCND) Consumer Nutrition
    Hot Line 1-800-366-1655

Canada

Canadian Celiac Disease Association
    6519B Mississauga Road
    Mississauga, Ontario L5N 1A6
    1-800-363-7296 or (905) 567-7195

National Institute of Nutrition
    302–265 Carling Ave.
    Ottawa, Ontario
    K1S 2E1
    (613) 235-3355
    Fax: (613) 235-7032

Links from sarahealth.com

For more information about disease prevention and wellness, visit me online at www.sarahealth.com, where you will find over three hundred links—including these—related to your good health and wellness.

- International Foundation for Functional GI Disorders (IFGD): information on IBS, GERD, abdominal and pelvic pain, bowel incontinence, and GI disorders. www.ifffgd.org
- Canadian Association of Gastroenterology. www.cag.ucalgary.ca
- The Helicobacter Foundation. www.helico.com
- GERD Information Resource Center: targets both a general audience and medical professionals; information about prevention, causes, symptoms, treatment, and medication. www.gerd.com
- Understanding GERD: patient education. www.acg.gi.org/gerd/gerdmain.htm

- PharmInfo: GERD and Heartburn Information Center; articles, news, drugs. www.pharminfo.com/disease/gerd/gerd_info.html

- GI Discussion Group: dissemination of medical bulletins and discussion of new research. www.pharminfo.com/disease/gastro/gast_lst.html #gastro-ehlb

- IBS Web Page and Resource Center: information, illustrations, book reviews, and links. www.healingwell.com/ibs/

- The IBS Page: information on constipation, diarrhea, and gas. www.panix.com/~ibs/

- Irritable Bowel Care: articles, resources, glossary, physician finder, and chat. www.irritablebowelcare.com

- Gallstones: general information, causes, and cures. www.niddk.nih.gov/Gallstones/Gallstones.html

- IBS Self-Help Group: www.ibsgroup.org

- Heartburn Help: a good source of information on heartburn and GERD. www.heartburnhelp.com

- Chinese Approach to IBS. http://acupunture.com/Acup/IBS.htm

- Center Watch: clinical trials for IBS. www.centerwatch.com/studies/cat90.htm

- Peptic Ulcer Information (from mediconsult.com). www.mediconsult.com/peptic/

- No Milk: information on lactose maldigestion, milk allergies, and casein intolerance. www.nomilk.com

- Canadian Celiac Association. www.celiac.ca

- The Celiac Disease Foundation. www.celiac.org

- The Gluten Intolerance Group of North America. www.gluten.net/default.htm

- The 24-Hour Acid Control Center: great source of information for frequent heartburn sufferers. www.acidcontrol.com

- Shwachman Syndrome: information about Shwachman Syndrome, a rare digestive disorder, with resources for patient-to-patient support. http://open.entry.com/medreal/shwach.htm

- Three Rivers Endoscopy Center: medical website about digestive health with emphasis on prevention. www.gihealth.com

- Crohn's, Ulcerative Colitis, and IBD Pages: with interactive message board. http://qurlyjoe.bu.edu/cduchome.html

- Crohn's and Colitis Foundation of America. www.ccfa.org

- The Culinary Couple's Creative Colitis Cookbook: one hundred low-fiber, nondairy recipes for those on restricted diets due to Crohn's or ulcerative colitis. www.colitiscookbook.com

- National Institute of Diabetes and Digestive Kidney Disease. www.niddk.nih.gov/

- Colon Cancer Alliance: news, research, advocacy, screening tips, and helpful organizations list. www.ccalliance.com

- American Cancer Society's Colorectal Cancer Overview: information on prevention, symptoms, treatment, drugs, and FAQs. www.3.cancer.org/cancerinfo/documents/overview/col ooover.asp?ct=10

- Colorectal Cancer Association of Canada.
  www.ccas-accc.ca
- American Digestive Health Foundation Colorectal
  Cancer Fact Sheet.
  www.gastro.org/drdan-colc.html
- Cancer Family Registries: contains two international
  family registries focusing on breast, ovarian, and
  colorectal cancer, offering families the opportunity to
  participate in important research studies.
  www.dccps.ims.nci.nih.gov/EGRP/cfr.html
- Medicine Online: Colon Cancer Information Library.
  www.meds.com/colon.colon.html
- Colon Connections: general information, news, and
  articles; screening and treatment facts. Both
  conventional and alternative approaches outlined.
  http://rattler.cameron.edu/colon/
- Colon Cancer Alliance Buddies Program: links survivors,
  caregivers, family, and friends for sharing and
  support. www.ccalliance.org/support/buddy.html
- Colon Cancer Risk Index: a questionnaire to calculate
  risk, put out by the Harvard Center for Cancer
  Prevention. www.hsph.harvard.edu/colonrisk/
- Colorado Health Net Cancer Center–Colon and Rectal
  Cancer Library: news, articles, useful links.
  www.coloradohealthnet.org/cancer/colon/colon_lib.html
- National Cancer Institute's Colon Cancer Site: very
  comprehensive information from the National
  Institutes of Health.
  http://cancernet.nci.nih.gov/Cancer_Types/Colon_And
  _Rectal_Cancer.shtml

- Atlas of Endoscopy: endoscopic views from the esophagus, stomach, duodenum, ERCP, and colon. http://home.t-online.de/home/afreytag/index.htm
- Crohn's and Colitis Foundation of America. www.ccfa.org

Bibliography

Adamek, R.J., Opferkuch, W., and Wegener, M. "Modified short-term triple therapy—ranitidine, clarithromycin, and metronidazole—for cure of Helicobacter pylori infection," *American Journal of Gastroenterology* (1995 Jan), 90(1):168–9.

Anvari, M., Allen, C., and Borm, A. "Laparoscopic Nissen fundoplication is a satisfactory alternative to long-term omeprazole therapy." *British Journal of Surgery* (1995 Jul), 82(7):938–42.

Arvanitakis, C., et al. "Cisapride and ranitidine in the treatment of gastro-oesophageal reflux disease—a comparative randomized double-blind trial." *Alimentary Pharmacology & Therapeutics* (1993), 7:635–41.

Atanassoff, P.G., Brull, S.J., Weiss, B.M., Landefeld, K., Alon, E., and Rohling, R. "The time course of gastric pH changes induced by omeprazole and ranitidine: A twenty-four hour dose-response study." *Alimentary Pharmacology & Therapeutics*

Bardhan, K.D., Ahlberg, J., Hislop, W.S., Lindholmer, C., Long, R.G., Morgan, A.G., Sjostedt, S., Smith, P.M., Stig, R., and Wormsley, K.G. "Rapid healing of gastric ulcers with lansoprazole." *Alimentary Pharmacology & Therapeutics* (1994 April), 8(2):215–20.

Bardhan, K.D., Hawkey, C.J., Long, R.G., Morgan, A.G., Wormsley, K.G., Moules, I.K., and Brocklebank, D. "Lansoprazole versus ranitidine for the treatment of reflux oesophagitis." UK Lansoprazole Clinical Research Group. *Alimentary Pharmacology & Therapeutics* (1995 Apr) 9(2):145–51.

Bell, G.D., Powell, K.U., Burridge, S.M., Bowden, A.F., Atoyebi, W., Bolton, G.H., Jones, P.H., Brown, C., Blum, A.L., Adami, B., and Bouzo, M.H. "Effect of cisapride on relapse of esophagitis: A multinational, placebo-controlled trial in patients healed with an antisecretory drug." *Digestive Diseases and Sciences* (1993) 38(3):551–560.

Blum, A.L., and Huijghebaert, S. "Long-term treatment of gastro-esophageal reflux disease: Experience with cisapride." *Today's Therapeutic Trends* (1994) 11(4):219–47.

Bortolotti, M., Cucchiara, S., Sarti, P., Brunelli, F., Mazza, M., Bagnato, F., and Barbara, L. "Comparison between the effects of neostigmine and ranitidine on interdigestive gastroduodenal motility of patients with gastroparesis." *Digestion* (1995), 56(2):96–9.

Carvalhinhos, A., Fidalgo, P., Freire, A., and Matos, L. "Cisapride compared with ranitidine in the treatment of functional dyspepsia." *European Journal of Gastroenterology and Hepatology* (1995 May), 7(5):411–17.

Castell, D.O. "Long-term management of GERD: The pill, the knife, or the endoscope?" *Gastrointestinal Endoscopy* (1994 Mar–Apr), 40(2 Pt 1):252–3.

Castell, D.O. "Introduction to pathophysiology of gastroesophageal reflux." In *Gastroesophageal Reflux Disease,* Castell, D.O., Wu, W.C., and Ott, D.J., eds. Mount Kisco, New York: Futura Publishing Company Inc., 1985; pp. 3–9.

Chal, K.L., Stacey, J.H., and Sacks, G.E. "The effect of ranitidine on symptom relief and quality of life of patients with gastro-oesophageal reflux disease." *British Journal of Clinical Practice* (1995 Mar–Apr), 49(2):73–7.

Cloud, M.L., and Offen, W.W. "Nizatidine versus placebo in gastro-oesophageal reflux disease: A 6-week, multicentre, randomised, double-blind comparison." Nizatidine Gastroesophageal Reflux Disease Study Group. *British Journal of Clinical Practice Symposium Supplement* (1994 Nov), 76:11–9.

Collen, M.J., Johnson, D.A., and Sheridan, M.J. "Basal acid output and gastric acid hypersecretion in gastroesophageal reflux disease. Correlation with ranitidine therapy." *Digestive Diseases and Sciences* (1994 Feb), 39(2):410–7.

Collen, M.J., and Strong, R.M. "Treatment of pyrosis does not insure adequate control of gastric acid reflux." *American Journal of Gastroenterology* (1995 Apr), 90(4):672–3.

Conference Reporter, Contemporary Issues in G.I. Motility Disorders. Special report from the 10th World Congress of Gastroenterology. "Convincing clinical results with motility drugs force re-evaluation of the management of GERD," Oct 2–7, 1994, Los Angeles, Calif.

Connelly, J.F. "Adjusting dosage intervals of intermittent intravenous ranitidine according to creatinine clearance: A cost-minimization analysis." *Hospital Pharmacy* (1994 Nov), 29(11):992, 996–8, 1001.

Dakkak, M., Jones, B.P., Scott, M.G., Tooley, P.J., and Bennett, J.R. "Comparing the efficacy of cisapride and ranitidine in oesophagitis: A double-blind, parallel group study in general practice." *British Journal of Clinical Practice* (1994 Jan–Feb), 48(1):10–14.

Dashe, Alfred M., MD., F.A.C.P., *The Man's Health Sourcebook*. Los Angeles: Lowell House, 1996.

de Boer, W., Driessen, W., Jansz, A., and Tytgat, G. "Effect of acid suppression on efficacy of treatment for Helicobacter pylori infection." *Lancet* (1995 Apr 1), 345(8953):817–20.

Dehbashi, N. "Effect of triple therapy or amoxycillin plus omeprazole or amoxycillin plus tinidazole plus omeprazole on duodenal ulcer healing, eradication of Helicobacter pylori, and prevention of ulcer relapse over a 1-year follow-up period: A prospective, randomized, controlled study." *American Journal of Gastroenterology* (1995 Sep.), 90(9):1419–23.

Dworkin, B.M., Rosenthal, W.S., Casellas, A.R., Girolomo, R., Lebovics, E., Freeman, S., and Clark, S.B. "Open label study of long-term effectiveness of cisapride in patients with idiopathic gastroparesis." *Digestive Diseases and Sciences* (1994)7:1395–8.

Fehr, H.F. "Risk factors, co-medication, and concomitant diseases: their influence on the outcome of therapy with cisapride." *Scandinavian Journal of Gastroenterology* (1993)28 Suppl 195:40–6.

Fennerty, M.B. "Helicobacter pylori." *Archives of Internal Medicine* (1994)154:721–7.

Fisher, R.S., and Ogorek, C.P. "Management of gastroesophageal reflux disease, part one: Pathogenesis, symptoms, and diagnosis." *Practical Gastroenterology,* (1994)18(9):21–2,24–6,32–5.

Fraser, R.J., Horowitz, M., Maddox, A.F., and Dent, J. "Postprandial antropyloroduodenal motility and gastric emptying in gastroparesis — effects of cisapride." *Gut* (1994 Feb), 35(2):172–8.

Fumagalli, I., and Hammer, B. "Cisapride versus metoclopramide in the treatment of functional dyspepsia: A double-blind comparative trial." *Scandinavian Journal of Gastroenterology* (1994 Jan), 29(1):33–7.

Galmiche, J.P., et al. "Double-blind comparison of cisapride and cimetidine in treatment of reflux esophagitis." *Digestive Diseases and Sciences* (1990), 35(5):649–55.

Geldof, H., Hazelhoff, B., and Otten, M.H. "Two different dose regimens of cisapride in the treatment of reflux oesophagitis: A double-blind comparison with ranitidine." *Alimentary Pharmacology & Therapeutics* (1993), 7:409–15.

Graham, K.S., Malaty, H., el-Zimaity, H.M., Genta, R.M., Cole, R.A., al-Assi, M.T., Yousfi, M.M., Neil, G.A., and Graham, D.Y. "Variability with omeprazole-amoxicillin combinations for treatment of Helicobacter pylori infection." *American Journal of Gastroenterology* (1995 Sep), 90(9):1415–18.

Halter, F., Miazza, B., and Brignoli, R. "Cisapride or cimetidine in the treatment of functional dyspepsia: Results of a double-blind, randomized, Swiss multicentre study." *Scandinavian Journal of Gastroenterology* (1994 Jul), 29(7):618–23.

Hausken, T., and Berstad, A. "Wide gastric antrum in patients with non-ulcer dyspepsia: effect of cisapride." *Scandinavian Journal of Gastroenterology* (1992), 27:427–32.

Heiselman, D.E., Hulisz, D.T., Fricker, R., Bredle, D.L., Black, L.D. "Randomized comparison of gastric pH control with intermittent and continuous intravenous infusion of famotidine in ICU patients." *American Journal of Gastroenterology* (1995 Feb), 90(2):277–9.

"Helicobacter pylori: A randomized trial employing 'optimal' dosing." *American Journal of Gastroenterology* (1995 Sep), 90(9):1407–10.

Hickner, J.M. "Ranitidine and GERD." *Journal of Family Practice* (1995 Aug), 41(2):186–7.

Hillman, A.L. "Economic analysis of alternative treatments for persistent gastro-oesophageal reflux disease." *Scandinavian Journal of Gastroenterology Supplement* (1994), 201:98–102.

Hislop, Gregory T., M.D.C.M., "The role of nutrition in
    the prevention of cancer." *Canadian Journal of CME,*
    (1995 March), 111–118.

Holtmann, G., et al. "Dyspepsia in healthy blood donors:
    Pattern of symptoms and association with
    Helicobacter pylori." *Digestive Diseases and Sciences*
    (1994 May), 39(5):1090–8.

James, O.F., and Parry-Billings, K.S. "Comparison of
    omeprazole and histamine H2-receptor antagonists in
    the treatment of elderly and young patients with
    reflux oesophagitis." *Age and Ageing* (1994 Mar),
    23(2):121–6.

Janisch, H.D., Huttemann, W., and Bouzo, M.H.,
    "Cisapride versus ranitidine in the treatment of reflux
    esophagitis." *Hepato-gastroenterology* (1988), 35:125–7.

Jian, R., et al. "Symptomatic, radionuclide and therapeutic
    assessment of chronic idiopathic dyspepsia: A double-
    blind placebo-controlled evaluation of cisapride."
    Digestive Disease Science (1989), 5:657–64.

Kellow, J.E., Cowan, H., Shuter, B., Riley, J.W., Lunzer,
    M.R., Eckstein, R.P., Hoschl, R., and Lam, S.K.
    "Efficacy of cisapride therapy in functional
    dyspepsia." *Alimentary Pharmacology & Therapeutics*
    (1995 Apr), 9(2):153–60.

Kimmig, J. "Treatment and prevention of relapse of mild
    oesophagitis with omeprazole and cisapride:
    Comparison of two strategies." *Alimentary
    Pharmacology & Therapeutics* (1995 Jun), 9(3):281–6.

Klinkenberg-Knol, E.C., Festen, H.P., Jansen, J.B., Lamers, C.B., Nelis, F., Snel, P., Luckers, A., Dekkers, C.P., Havu, N., and Meuwissen, S.G. "Long-term treatment with omeprazole for refractory reflux esophagitis: Efficacy and safety." *Annals of Internal Medicine* (1994 Aug 1), 121(3):161–7.

Labenz, J., Leverkus, F., and Borsch, G. "Omeprazole plus amoxicillin for cure of Helicobacter pylori infection: Factors influencing the treatment success." *Scandinavian Journal of Gastroenterology* (1994 Dec), 29(12):1070–5.

Labenz, J., Ruhl, G.H., Bertrams, J., and Borsch, G. "Effective treatment after failure of omeprazole plus amoxycillin to eradicate Helicobacter pylori infection in peptic ulcer disease." *Alimentary Pharmacology & Therapeutics* (1994 Jun), 8(3):323–7.

Lepoutre, L., et al. "Healing of grade-II and III oesophagitis through motility stimulation with cisapride." *Digestion* (1990), 45:109–14.

Lockhart, S.P. "Clinical review of lansoprazole." *British Journal of Clinical Practice Symposium Supplement* (1994 May–Jun), 75:48–55; discussion, 56–7.

Louw, J.A., Lucke, W., Jaskiewicz, K., Lastovica, A.J., Winter, T.A., Marks, I.N. "Helicobacter pylori eradication in the African setting, with special reference to reinfection and duodenal ulcer recurrence." *Gut* (1995 Apr), 36(4):544–7.

Lux, G., Katschinski, M., Ludwig, S., Lederer, P., Ellermann, A., and Domschke, W. "The effect of cisapride and metoclopramide on human digestive and interdigestive antroduodenal motility." *Scandinavian Journal of Gastroenterology* (1994 Dec), 29(12):1105–10.

Maleev, A., et al. "Cisapride and cimetidine in the treatment of erosive esophagitis." *Hepato-gastoenterology* (1990), 37:403–7.

Malkoff, M.D., Ponzillo, J.J., Myles, G.L., Gomez, C.R., and Cruz-Flores, S. "Sinus arrest after administration of intravenous metoclopramide." *Annals of Pharmacotherary* (1995 Apr), 29(4):381–3.

Markowsky, S.J., and Santeiro, M.L. "Automatic therapeutic substitution: cost savings with intravenous push famotidine." *Annals of Pharmacotherary* (1995 Mar), 29(3):316.

Marks, R.D., Richter, J.E., Rizzo, J., Koehler, R.E., Spenney, J.G., Mills, T.P., and Champion, G. "Omeprazole versus H2-receptor antagonists in treating patients with peptic stricture and esophagitis." *Gastroenterology* (1994 Apr), 106(4):907–15.

Mason, Michael. "Forget Stress and Spicy Foods: The Real Culprit May Be Just a Kiss Away." (1994) *Health* 12(1):1–15

Mavromichalis, I., Zaramboukas, T., and Giala, M.M. "Migraine of gastrointestinal origin." *European Journal of Pediatrics* (1995 May), 154(5):406–10.

McCallum, R.W. "Cisapride for the treatment of nocturnal heartburn in patients with gastroesophageal reflux disease." *Today's Therapeutic Trends* (1994), 11(4):187–201.

Merki, H.S., and Wilder-Smith, C.H. "Do continuous infusions of omeprazole and ranitidine retain their effect with prolonged dosing?" *Gastroenterology* (1994 Jan), 106(1):60–4.

NIH Consensus Statement. "Helicobacter pylori in peptic ulcer disease." (1994), 12(1):1–15.

"Omeprazole vs. ranitidine for prevention of relapse in reflux oesophagitis: A controlled double-blind trial of their efficacy and safety." *Gut* (1994 May), 35(5):590–8.

"Open label study of long-term effectiveness of cisapride in patients with idiopathic gastroparesis." *Digestive Diseases and Sciences* (1994 Jul), 39(7):1395–8.

Orihata, M., and Sarna, S.K. "Contractile mechanisms of action of gastroprokinetic agents: Cisapride, metoclopramide, and domperidone." *American Journal of Physiology* (1994 Apr), 266(4 Pt 1):G665–76.

Orr, John. "Another man's poison." *Diabetes Dialogue*, (Spring 1996), 43, (1).

Orr, W.C. "The role of cisapride in the treatment of gastroesophageal reflux." In *Gastrointestinal Dysmotility: Focus on cisapride*, Heading, R.C., and Wood, J.D., eds. New York: Raven Press Ltd., 1992, pp.141–7.

————. "Upper Gastrointestinal Motor Functioning: A Physiologic Overview." *The Consultant Pharmacist* (1994), (Suppl A):4–13.

Park, K.N., Hahm, J.S., and Kim, H.J. "Pharmacological effects of metronidazole+tetracycline+bismuth subcitrate in Helicobacter pylori–related gastritis and peptic ulcer disease." *European Journal of Gastroenterology & Hepatology* (1994 Dec), 6 Suppl 1:S103–7.

Patient Information. The National Digestive Diseases Information Clearinghouse (NDDIC), a service of the National Institute of Diabetes and Digestive and Kidney Diseases, part of the National Institutes of Health, under the U.S. Public Health Service. 1996, National Digestive Diseases Information Clearinghouse, Licensed to Medical Strategies, Inc.

Pedrazzoli, J. Jr., Magalhaes, A.F., Ferraz, J.G., Trevisan, M., and De Nucci, G. "Triple therapy with sucralfate is not effective in eradicating Helicobacter pylori and does not reduce duodenal ulcer relapse rates." *American Journal of Gastroenterology* (1994 Sep), 89(9):1501–4.

Pipkin, G., and Mills, J.G. "Treatment of nonsteroidal anti-inflammatory drug–associated gastric and duodenal damage. Efficacy of antisecretory drugs and mucosal protective compounds." *Digestive Diseases* (1995 Jan), 13 Suppl 1:75–88.

"Predictive factors of the long-term outcome in gastro-oesophageal reflux disease: Six-year follow-up of 107 patients." *Gut* (1994 Jan), 35(1):8–14.

Rabeneck, L."Long-term treatment of erosive esophagitis with omeprazole: does it work?" *Gastroenterology* (1995 Feb), 108(2):613–4.

"Rapid eradication of Helicobacter pylori infection." *Alimentary Pharmacology & Therapeutics* (1995 Feb), 9(1):41–6.

Reekie, W.D., and Buxton, M.J. "Cost-effectiveness as a guide to pricing a new pharmaceutical product." *South Africa Medical Journal* (1994 Jul), 84(7):421–3.

Rezende-Filho, J. et al. "Cisapride stimulates antral motility and decreases biliary reflux in patients with severe dyspepsia." *Digestive Diseases and Sciences* (1989), 7:1057–62.

Riezzo, G., Cucchiara, S., Chiloiro, M., Minella, R., Guerra, V., and Giorgio, I. "Gastric emptying and myoelectrical activity in children with nonulcer dyspepsia: Effect of cisapride." *Digestive Diseases and Sciences* (1995 Jul), 40(7):1428–34.

Rosenthal, M. Sara. *Managing Your Diabetes*. Canada: Macmillan, 1998.

———. *The Gastrointestinal Sourcebook*. Lincolnwood, Ill.: NTC/Contemporary Books, 1998.

———. *Women and Depression*. Lincolnwood, Ill.: NTC/Contemporary Books, 1998.

Schindlbeck, N.E., Klauser, A.G., Voderholzer, W.A., and Muller-Lissner, S.A. "Empiric therapy for gastroesophageal reflux disease." *Archives of Internal Medicine* (1995, Sep 11), 155(16):1808–12.

Shintani, S., Shiigai, T., Tsuchiya, K., and Kikuchi, M. "Hyperventilation alternating with apnea in neuroleptic malignant syndrome associated with metoclopramide and cisapride." *Journal of Neurological Science* (1995 Feb), 128(2):232–3.

Sobhani, I., Chastang, C., De Korwin, J.D., Lamouliatte, H., Megraud, F., Guerre, J., and Elouaer-Blanc, L. "Antibiotic versus maintenance therapy in the prevention of duodenal ulcer recurrence: Results of a multicentric double-blind randomized trial." *Gastroenterology & Clinical Biology* (1995 Mar), 19(3):252–8.

Stubberod, A., Glise, H., Hallerback, B., and Solhaug, J.H. "The effect of cisapride and ranitidine as monotherapies and in combination in the treatment of uncomplicated gastric ulceration." *Scandinavian Journal of Gastroenterology* (1995 Feb), 30(2):106–10.

Sullivan, T.J., Reese., J.H., Jauregui, L., Miller, K., Levine, L., and Bachmann, K.A. "Short report: A comparative study of the interaction between antacid and H2-receptor antagonists." *Alimentary Pharmacology & Therapeutics* (1994 Feb), 8(1):123–6.

Svendsen, L.B., Ross, C., Knigge, U., Frederiksen, H.J., Graversen, P., Kjaergard, J., Luke, M., Stimpel, H., and Sparso, B.H. "Cimetidine as an adjuvant treatment in colorectal cancer: A double-blind, randomized pilot study." *Diseases of the Colon and Rectum* (1995 May), 38(5):514–8.

Toussaint, J. et al. "Healing and prevention of relapse of reflux by cisapride." *Gut* (1991), 32:1280–5.

Tofflemire, Jacqui. "Celiac disease." *Diabetes Dialogue* (1997 Spring), 44,(1).

Tytgat, G.N., Blum, A.L., and Verlinden, M. "Prognostic factors for relapse and maintenance treatment with cisapride in gastro-oesophageal reflux disease." *Alimentary Pharmacology & Therapeutics* (1995 Jun), 9(3):271–80.

Tytgat, G.N.J. "Prognostic factors affecting the duration of remission of gastro-oesophageal reflux disease." *Journal of Drug Development* (1993), 5 Suppl 2:21–5.

Veldhuyzen van Zanten, S.J.O., et al. "Helicobacter pylori infection as a cause of gastritis, duodenal ulcer, gastric cancer, and non-ulcer dyspepsia: A systematic overview," *Canadian Medical Association Journal* (1994, Jan 15), 150(2):177–185.

Wagner, B., and Nagata, M. "Oral ranitidine as stress ulcer prophylaxis: Serum concentrations and cost comparisons." *Critical Care Medicine* (1994 Jan), 22(1):177–8.

Walan, A., and Eriksson, S. "Long-term consequences with regard to clinical outcome and cost-effectiveness of episodic treatment with omeprazole or ranitidine for healing of duodenal ulcer." *Scandinavian Journal of Gastroenterology Supplement* (1994), 201:91–7.

Walsh, J.H., et al. "The treatment of Helicobacter pylori infection in the management of peptic ulcer disease." *New England Journal of Medicine* (1995, Oct 12)984–991.

Yousfi, M.M., el-Zimaity, H.M., al-Assi, M.T., Cole, R.A., Genta, R.M., Graham, D.Y. "Metronidazole, omeprazole, and clarithromycin: An effective combination therapy for Helicobacter pylori infection." *Alimentary Pharmacology & Therapeutics* (1995 Apr), 9(2):209–12.

Yousfi, M.M., Neil, G.A., and Graham, D.Y. "Variability with omeprazole-amoxicillin combinations for treatment of Helicobacter pylori infection." *American Journal of Gastroenterology* (1995 Sep), 90(9):1415–8.

Index